The Lost Herbal Medicine Bible

How to Craft Essential Oils, Tinctures, Infusions, and Antibiotics from Soil to Soul

Simon Jr. Jackson

Table of Contents

Introduction 4

   The Importance of Herbal Medicine 4

   A Note on Sustainability and Ethical Harvesting 5

Chapter 1: The Foundations of Herbal Medicine 7

   Historical Perspective 7

   Modern-day Relevance and Revival 11

Chapter 2: Setting Up Your Herbal Garden **14**

   Choosing the Right Location 15

   Soil, Sunlight, and Water Needs 19

   Common Herbs and Their Growing Conditions 22

Chapter 3: Essential Tools for the Herbalist **25**

   Basic Tools and Equipment 26

   Safety Protocols in Handling and Storage 29

Chapter 4: Crafting Essential Oils **33**

   Introduction to Essential Oils 34

   Extraction Methods 38

   Storing and Using Essential Oils Safely 43

Chapter 5: The Art of Making Tinctures **48**

   What are Tinctures? 49

   Tincturing Process 51

   Uses and Dosages 56

Chapter 6: Brewing Herbal Infusions **59**

   Understanding Infusions and Decoctions 60

   Techniques and Ratios 63

   Popular Herbal Infusions and Their Benefits 67

Chapter 7: Antibiotics from Nature **70**

A Brief History of Antibiotics 71

Herbal Alternatives to Common Antibiotics...73

Chapter 8: Harvesting and Drying Your Herbs **77**

Best Times and Methods for Harvesting 78

Drying Techniques...82

Storing Dried Herbs 85

Chapter 9: Real-Life Applications and Case Studies **88**

Personal Experiences with Herbal Medicine 88

Clinical Insights: What the Research Says 91

Appendix A: Glossary of Herbal Terms **93**

Appendix B: Herb Profiles **96**

Conclusion **108**

Bonus **109**

Introduction

The Importance of Herbal Medicine

Herbal medicine, or phytotherapy, is as ancient as human civilization. For as long as humans have walked the Earth, they've turned to flora for relief and cures. This ancient practice has its roots in observation and tradition. Our earliest ancestors noted how animals would consume specific plants when sick, intuitively aware of their medicinal properties. This observation eventually gave rise to traditional medicinal systems like Ayurveda in India and Traditional Chinese Medicine in China, each with a rich pharmacopeia of plants and herbs. Even the word 'drug' comes from the Old Dutch word 'droog,' meaning 'to dry,' hinting at the practice of drying herbs for medicinal purposes.

Modern medicine has provided a plethora of benefits, including vaccines, surgical procedures, and life-saving drugs. But this boon also presents a dilemma—the 'pill for every ill' mentality. The prevalent mindset in modern healthcare often ignores lifestyle and environmental factors, focusing instead on symptom management via pharmaceuticals. While useful for acute conditions, this approach has led to over-prescription. For example, the misuse of antibiotics has contributed to antibiotic resistance, a grave concern for global public health. Similarly, the rise of opioid prescriptions for pain management has contributed to the devastating opioid crisis.

Although herbal medicine is rooted in ancient tradition, modern science increasingly validates its effectiveness. Willow bark, rich in salicylic acid, led to the creation of aspirin, a drug widely used for pain relief and cardiovascular health. The anti-malarial drug quinine is derived from the bark of the cinchona tree. Furthermore, ongoing research is studying herbs like turmeric, known for its anti-inflammatory properties; garlic, famed for its antibacterial capabilities; and even plants like cannabis, under investigation for a wide range of medicinal applications. Such scientific validation is vital in positioning herbal medicine as a complement to synthetic pharmaceuticals.

When administered correctly, herbal medicine is generally considered safe and often comes with fewer side effects compared to its synthetic counterparts. This safety makes herbal medicine an attractive option for chronic conditions and preventive health. Additionally, herbal remedies are usually more cost-effective. While the pharmaceutical industry often charges astronomical sums for patented drugs, many medicinal herbs can be grown in your backyard or foraged responsibly from the wild. However, it's essential to acknowledge the importance of dosage and potential interactions with other medications you may be taking.

Beyond the physical benefits, herbal medicine offers a psychological and spiritual boon: a reconnection with the natural world. The act of foraging, growing, and preparing herbal remedies can be deeply enriching. It enables us to step away from the chaos of modern life and re-establish a link with the rhythms and cycles of nature, thereby benefiting not just our bodies but also our mental and emotional well-being.

As healthcare systems evolve, we're witnessing a shift towards more integrative and holistic approaches. These perspectives align well with the principles of herbal medicine, which often focuses on treating the root causes of ailments rather than merely addressing symptoms. Given the rising costs of healthcare and the over-reliance on pharmaceuticals, herbal medicine is well-positioned to play a significant role in the future of healthcare.

Herbal medicine has long been a cornerstone of human healthcare and is increasingly validated by modern science. It's a field that doesn't just treat symptoms but aims to harmonize the body and treat the root causes of ailments. It provides a unique opportunity to reconnect with the natural world, offering healing that is both physical and spiritual. As we move into the future, herbal medicine will undoubtedly play an increasingly vital role in the landscape of global healthcare.

A Note on Sustainability and Ethical Harvesting

One of the most profound aspects of herbal medicine is its rootedness in nature, emphasizing the symbiotic relationship between humans and the Earth. But this connection also brings forth a responsibility—to ensure that our quest for health and well-being does not come at the expense of the environment. We are but a thread in the intricate web of life, and our actions have far-reaching implications.

Herbs like Goldenseal and American Ginseng have become endangered due to overharvesting. The increasing popularity of herbal medicine has led to a surge in demand, often fulfilled by irresponsible harvesting methods. Overharvesting can lead to soil degradation, habitat destruction, and a decline in biodiversity. It's a paradox: the very plants that offer us healing could be at risk of extinction if we don't adopt sustainable practices. Practicing ethical harvesting is more than just taking what you need; it's about understanding the plant's life cycle, its role in the ecosystem, and how your actions will impact future growth. Some general guidelines include never taking more than 10-20% of a plant population, avoiding harvesting from endangered species, and replanting seeds when possible. It's also essential to have proper identification skills to ensure that you're not mistakenly harvesting a protected or endangered species.

One way to circumvent the risks of overharvesting is to cultivate your own medicinal herbs. This not only ensures a personal supply but also reduces pressure on wild populations. However, cultivation comes with its own set of responsibilities, like avoiding the use of synthetic pesticides and fertilizers that can harm the environment. Organic, permaculture-based methods offer a sustainable alternative that can yield potent medicinal plants while enhancing soil health and biodiversity. Before you set out with your basket and shears, be aware that harvesting plants—even weeds—from public lands often requires a permit. In some cases, it's illegal to harvest particular plants that are considered endangered or protected. Always do your research on local regulations and obtain necessary permissions to avoid legal consequences.

Sustainability is a community effort. The more people are educated about the importance of ethical harvesting and sustainable practices, the greater the impact we can make. Workshops, community gardens, and social media platforms can serve as powerful tools for raising awareness and teaching essential skills. By fostering a community of responsible herbalists, we can help preserve these ancient practices for future generations.

Sustainable, ethical harvesting is not just a side note in the practice of herbal medicine; it's a crucial component. It reflects a holistic understanding that our health and the health of our planet are inextricably linked. The herbs we seek for healing offer their medicine willingly, but we must reciprocate with respect and care to ensure that these plants—and the ecosystems they inhabit— continue to flourish for years to come.

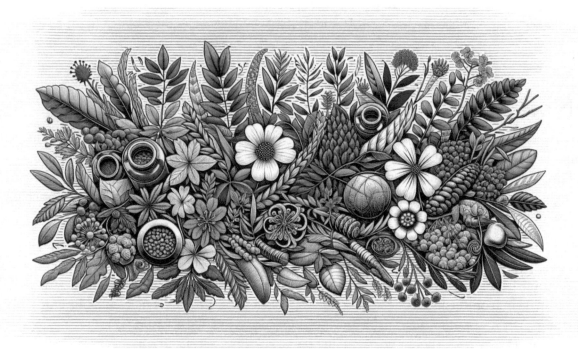

Chapter 1: The Foundations of Herbal Medicine

Welcome to Chapter 1 of our herbal medicine journey, where we're going to dig deep into the rich soil of knowledge about the foundations of herbal medicine. Imagine this chapter as the sturdy roots of a towering oak tree; it's where our herbal wisdom begins to take root and grow.

In this chapter, we'll embark on a captivating exploration of two essential subtopics:

Just like uncovering a treasure chest of ancient scrolls, we'll delve into the historical tapestry of herbal medicine. You'll get to know the remarkable stories of healers and herbalists from bygone eras, who relied on the power of nature to cure ailments. It's a journey back in time, and we'll uncover the fascinating roots of herbal medicine that connect us to our ancestors.

Now, let's fast-forward to the present day. We'll shine a light on how herbal medicine isn't just a relic of the past; it's a vibrant and thriving practice in our contemporary world. We'll explore how traditional wisdom meets modern science, and how herbal remedies are finding their place in today's wellness landscape. It's like discovering a hidden gem in your own backyard.

Throughout this chapter, we'll be your guides, walking alongside you as we unravel the past and embrace the present of herbal medicine. So, put on your herbalist hat, grab a cup of your favorite herbal tea, and let's dive into the enthralling world of herbal healing. Get ready to unearth the secrets that plants have been whispering to us for centuries.

Historical Perspective

Imagine, if you will, a time before aspirin bottles lined the shelves of pharmacies, before the convenience of antibiotics or the magic of anesthetic drugs. Picture a world where people relied solely on what nature provided them. This was the cradle of herbal medicine, a practice as old as human history itself. The intertwined roots of plants and human health go deep, digging back into prehistoric times when early humans would have relied on trial and error, figuring out that some leaves could heal and others could harm.

Isn't it fascinating to think about the first person who discovered that chewing on a willow bark could alleviate pain? They didn't have a scientific journal to publish their findings or social media to share their discovery. Yet, this ancient wisdom passed down through generations, shaping the future of pain relief—literally laying the groundwork for what would one day become aspirin as we know it.

Throughout the annals of history, herbal medicine has been the cornerstone of healthcare in diverse civilizations. In ancient Egypt, texts like the Ebers Papyrus listed remedies for various ailments, many of which included herbs like garlic and juniper. Flash forward to Greece, where the renowned Hippocrates, often considered the father of modern medicine, laid down theories about the humoral system and the role of natural substances in balancing bodily fluids.

You might ask, how did the Chinese and Indian Ayurvedic traditions fit into all of this? Well, in a similar vein, these cultures had their own vast pharmacopeias. Acupuncture often gets the spotlight when discussing Chinese medicine, but herbs have been the unsung heroes, doing the heavy lifting behind the scenes. In India, the use of herbs like Turmeric and Ashwagandha have been mentioned in Ayurvedic texts that date back thousands of years.

Now, let's hop on a ship and sail to the Middle Ages in Europe. Picture dark ages and plagues, a time when the line between medicine and magic seemed rather thin. Monasteries were the keepers of medicinal knowledge, carefully transcribing texts and cultivating herb gardens. It was also the time when Nicholas Culpeper, an English botanist and herbalist, wrote his "Complete Herbal," offering comprehensive information on the uses of different plants. This text was revolutionary because it made herbal medicine accessible to the common folk, stripping away the Latin jargon and elitism that had previously confined this knowledge to the clergy and educated class.

Let's fast-forward a bit to the Enlightenment, the age of reason, when herbal medicine faced an identity crisis. While some viewed it as unscientific folklore, others saw it as a treasure trove of untapped potential. Linnaeus' work in plant taxonomy gave a more structured framework for understanding herbs, which allowed researchers to study plants with a more scientific lens. The 19th century saw the birth of phytochemistry, the study of plant compounds, which led to the isolation of molecules like morphine from the opium poppy. It was a turning point that fueled the pharmaceutical revolution, giving rise to a whole new era of synthesized medicines.

You might be wondering, where does herbal medicine stand today amidst all this modern technology? You see, it's experiencing a revival, a renaissance if you will. As much as we've advanced in the realm of medicine, there's a growing recognition that synthetic drugs aren't the be-all and end-all. With antibiotic resistance on the rise and an increasing focus on personalized medicine, people are turning back to herbs, not just as alternative remedies but as complementary therapies. And this is not just a grassroots movement; even the scientific community is re-examining herbal medicines, fueled by cutting-edge research and clinical trials.

So what's the takeaway from this whirlwind tour of herbal medicine through the ages? It's that herbs have been our constant companions, their uses adapting and evolving, but their essence remaining the same—a natural extension of our world, offering remedies, relief, and resilience. The challenge and opportunity for us now lie in integrating this ancient wisdom with modern science in a way that respects the earth, prioritizes sustainability, and focuses on holistic well-being.

Ready to make this age-old tradition a part of your own health journey? Let's keep exploring together.

As we journey through the annals of time and space, let's set our sights on the indigenous peoples of North America. The Native Americans offer a unique perspective on herbal medicine, blending the physical, spiritual, and ecological into an intricate tapestry of healing. To truly understand Native American herbal medicine, you have to first grasp their holistic worldview. For them, health was not just the absence of disease; it was a state of harmony—between the body, the spirit, and Mother Earth. It was a symphony where each plant played a unique note.

Imagine walking through a forest with a Native American healer—known in various tribes as a shaman, medicine man, or medicine woman. You'd probably notice how the healer wouldn't just randomly pick plants. Instead, each herb was chosen with intention and reverence, often accompanied by rituals or prayers. They believed that each plant had a spirit, and acknowledging that spirit was an integral part of the healing process. A unique blend of spirituality and practicality, don't you think?

The indigenous knowledge about plants was incredibly detailed. From sage to cedar, tobacco to sweetgrass, each herb had a purpose. They used herbs for a range of needs: as antiseptics for wound healing, as remedies for common ailments like colds or digestive issues, and as psychoactive substances for spiritual rituals. Ever heard of echinacea? Native Americans were using it for boosting immunity long before it became a staple in modern health food stores.

One practice that's gaining contemporary attention is the ritual of smudging, which involves burning specific herbs like sage, cedar, or sweetgrass. Far from being a "trendy" activity, this ceremonial practice was used for purification and to establish a sacred space. And guess what? Recent scientific studies have found that burning sage can actually purify the air of harmful bacteria. In essence, tradition and science come full circle! The herbal wisdom of Native Americans didn't just stay within the confines of their communities. When European settlers arrived, they brought their own medical practices, but they also learned from Native Americans. Remember that the next time you're sipping on some chamomile tea to ease your nerves; chamomile was another plant used by Native Americans long before it became a European staple.

If there's one thing we should emulate from Native American herbal practices, it's their deep-rooted respect for the Earth. Sustainable harvesting was second nature to them. They understood the concept of taking only what you need and leaving enough for the plant to continue its life cycle. It was an intimate relationship, a give-and-take that ensured not just the survival but also the thriving of both parties. Today, as more people turn back to herbal medicine, it's crucial to approach it with a sense of reverence and responsibility. Just like the Native Americans, we must be cautious stewards of the Earth, honoring not just the utility but also the spirit of each plant.

The Native American perspective serves as a vivid reminder that herbal medicine is more than just a collection of remedies; it's a worldview, a way of life, and a tradition that spans millennia. As we continue to explore the broad spectrum of herbal medicine, let's carry forth the lessons learned from the Native Americans—lessons of harmony, sustainability, and the interconnectedness of all things.

Geronimo, the famed Apache leader, was not just a warrior but also known to be a skilled herbalist. He used indigenous herbs for healing various ailments among his people. Although the details of his herbal repertoire are not extensively documented, accounts suggest that he often employed native plants for respiratory conditions and gastrointestinal issues.

The annals of history are peppered with figures who turned to natural remedies, sometimes out of necessity and sometimes out of a profound respect for herbal medicine. Let's explore a few of these intriguing tales!

Yes, the very Hippocrates who gave us the Hippocratic Oath, which doctors still swear by today. Now, you'd think someone often referred to as the "Father of Medicine" would be all about the science and less about the herbs, right? Wrong! Hippocrates was a keen herbalist and is said to have had a collection of around 400 different types of herbs. One of his favorite remedies for pain and fever was willow bark—the very same substance that led to the development of aspirin. Talk about being ahead of his time!

Hildegard of Bingen was a German nun in the 12th century, but calling her just a nun would be doing her a disservice. She was a composer, a philosopher, and—you guessed it—a herbalist! Her written works on herbal medicine were groundbreaking for her time and were read and used long after she was gone. One of her go-to herbs was the humble lavender, which she recommended for everything from headaches to mental health. If Hildegard was around today, she'd probably be a fan of lavender essential oils!

Yes, the U.S. President Thomas Jefferson was a bit of an herbal enthusiast himself. Jefferson cultivated a variety of herbs in his Monticello garden, both for culinary and medicinal uses. One of his letters even mentions how he preferred using "the resources of the vegetable kingdom" for his headaches rather than relying on "noxious" minerals like mercury—quite sensible given what we now know about mercury poisoning!

You remember Nicholas Culpeper, the English botanist we talked about earlier, right? Well, he wasn't just an academic; he practiced what he preached. Culpeper was often at odds with the medical establishment of his day and offered free consultations using herbs. He even took his expertise onto the battlefield during the English Civil War, tending to wounded soldiers using his herbal preparations. Some say his own frequent illnesses, which he treated with herbs, were what motivated him to help others.

Isn't it fascinating to think that these titans of history, often celebrated for totally different achievements, also dabbled in the art of herbal healing? Whether it was out of necessity or driven by a deep respect for natural medicine, each found relief and resilience in the arms of Mother Nature. It's almost like they're whispering through the ages, reminding us that sometimes, the remedies we seek are growing right in our backyards—or at least, in the pages of a good herbal guidebook.

So, intrigued enough to give herbal medicine a shot in your own life? Trust me, you'd be in excellent company!

Modern-day Relevance and Revival

The pendulum of time swings, and here we are in the modern world, filled with gadgets, filled with science, filled with—pills? Yes, for a long time, modern medicine looked like a pharmaceutical catalog. However, the pendulum is swinging back, my friends. We're rediscovering what our ancestors knew instinctively: that Mother Nature is a wellspring of remedies, and herbal medicine is making a big, glorious comeback. So, grab a cup of your favorite herbal tea, and let's delve into how and why this is happening.

In this tech-driven world, you might wonder, "Why herbs?" The answer is simple: it works. But this isn't just grandma's old wisdom talking. Modern research is giving a nod to many herbal remedies that have been used for centuries. Turmeric, which has been a staple in Indian Ayurvedic medicine, is now being studied for its anti-inflammatory and anti-cancer properties. St. John's Wort, an old European remedy for mental health, is now recognized for its antidepressant qualities. The line between the so-called "alternative" and mainstream medicine is blurring, and that's a good thing.

Have you ever wondered why certain medications work wonders for some but fall flat for others?

That's because we're all unique, not just in our personalities but also in our biology. The one-size-fits-all approach is fading, making way for more personalized medicine. This is where herbal medicine shines. With a vast array of herbs at our disposal, finding a remedy that works uniquely for you has never been easier. Whether it's ginger tea for nausea or peppermint oil for migraines, there's probably an herb that fits you like a glove.

Let's face it, healthcare can be expensive. Even with insurance, the costs can be prohibitive. Herbal remedies offer a more affordable alternative. Plus, many herbs are easy to grow at home, reducing costs even further. A sprig of rosemary or thyme from your garden? That's practically free! The low barrier to entry makes herbal medicine incredibly accessible, and that's part of its modern-day appeal.

There's a certain empowerment in being able to take charge of your own health. The DIY culture has seeped into healthcare as well, with more people making their own tinctures, salves, and teas. The internet is flush with tutorials and recipes, transforming laypeople into at-home herbalists. If you've ever made your own chamomile tea to help you sleep or whipped up a lavender salve for stress relief, you're part of this revolution. Some people see herbal medicine and pharmaceuticals as opposing forces, but the truth is, they can work wonderfully together. Many healthcare providers now consider herbal history when prescribing medications, and some even recommend herbal supplements alongside traditional treatments. It's a holistic approach, taking the best of both worlds to give you the most comprehensive care possible. Herbal medicine is no longer just folk wisdom passed down through generations; it's becoming an academic subject. Various institutes and universities now offer certified courses in herbalism, pharmacognosy, and even Ayurveda and Traditional Chinese Medicine. This is crucial for standardizing and validating the practice, ensuring that the herbal remedies you use are both safe and effective.

Genomics is the study of all of a person's genes and their interactions. With advancements in this field, there's the exciting potential to match specific herbal remedies to individual genetic profiles.

Imagine a future where your herbal treatment plan is tailored not just to your symptoms, but to your very DNA!

The power of Instagram, right? One post about the benefits of ashwagandha or CBD oil, and suddenly it's the talk of the town. But it's not just hype. The wellness movement, fueled by social media, has made people more conscious of what they put into their bodies. This digital-age word-of-mouth has given herbal medicine a platform it never had before, making it accessible to a wider audience. It's like the Renaissance of herbal medicine, but with hashtags!

If there's one thing that modern society is waking up to, it's the importance of taking care of our planet. Synthetic drugs often involve processes that are harmful to the environment, not to mention the issue of pharmaceutical waste. Herbs? They're as green as it gets! More and more people are growing their own herbal gardens, and companies are investing in sustainable harvesting. It's a win-win situation for both your health and Mother Earth. In this age of global connectivity, it's not just goods and services that cross borders; knowledge does too. Traditions and practices once isolated to specific parts of the world are now being shared far and wide. Ever heard of Moringa? It's a plant native to parts of Africa and Asia, hailed as a "miracle tree" for its multiple health benefits. A decade ago, it was relatively unknown in the West. Today, it's everywhere—thanks to the internet and global trade. This fusion of herbal traditions from around the world enriches our collective knowledge and expands our healing arsenal.

Women have been the keepers of herbal wisdom for centuries, often serving as the family healers. Modern herbalism is picking up on this legacy, with a growing focus on herbs that address women's specific health needs. From raspberry leaf tea for menstrual discomfort to fenugreek for boosting milk supply in lactating mothers, herbs are gaining recognition as potent remedies for women's health issues. The conversation around mental health has evolved significantly in recent years. As we look for ways to manage stress, anxiety, and depression, herbal allies like St. John's Wort and Valerian root are increasingly making their way into the mainstream dialogue. Even adaptogens, herbs that help the body adapt to stress, like Ashwagandha and Holy Basil, are becoming popular for mental resilience.

Even in the realm of sports, athletes are turning to herbal supplements to enhance performance and recovery. Substances like Ginseng and Rhodiola Rosea are known for boosting stamina and reducing fatigue, helping athletes perform at their peak. And it's not just for the professionals; everyday fitness enthusiasts are also incorporating these herbal supplements into their routines.

As much as herbalism is a practice rooted in ancient wisdom, it's also embracing the advantages of technology. Apps and software that help identify plants, track symptoms, and even plan herbal gardens are becoming popular. These digital tools serve as a bridge between age-old practices and modern conveniences, making herbalism more accessible than ever. The culinary world is also getting a herbal makeover. Chefs and home cooks alike are discovering that herbs can do more than just season food; they can actually be the star of the dish, offering both flavor and health benefits. So the next time you add some rosemary to your roasted potatoes, know that you're not just making them tasty—you're making them healthier!

As herbal medicine gains traction, there's a growing need for regulation to ensure safety and efficacy. Some countries are beginning to recognize herbal medicine as a legitimate healthcare choice, and are implementing policies to regulate the practice, including standardizing the education of herbalists. This is an important step toward the integration of herbal and conventional medicine, ensuring that herbal remedies meet the same quality standards as pharmaceuticals. Last but not least, let's talk about the kiddos. As parents become more health-conscious, they're also becoming more hesitant to pump their children full of synthetic drugs for every little ailment. Herbs like chamomile for relaxation, echinacea for immune support, and peppermint for digestive issues are finding their way into children's health regimens. However, it's crucial to consult healthcare professionals when using herbs for children to ensure they are both effective and safe.

So, there you have it—a panoramic view of herbal medicine's burgeoning relevance in our lives today. It's a field in flux, shaped by trends and innovations but anchored in traditions that have stood the test of time. As you navigate your own health journey, consider how this ancient wisdom could complement the modern tools at your disposal.

It's a big herbal world out there, and we're all students. What are you curious about? What will you try next? Remember, the herbal path is as much about exploration and discovery as it is about healing.

Chapter 2: Setting Up Your Herbal Garden

If you've been nodding along through our historical journey and the modern-day revival of herbal medicine, you're probably tingling with excitement to start your own herbal haven. Imagine this: stepping into your garden, the air infused with the aromatic blend of rosemary, mint, and lavender. You pick a few sprigs here and there, not from the grocery store shelf, but right from the soil that you've nurtured. There's something almost magical about it, don't you think?

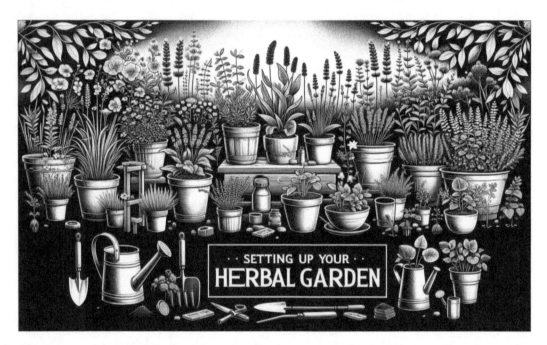

But hold on, eager herbalist! Before you start digging up your backyard or raiding the garden center, there are some essential things to consider. Trust me; a little planning will go a long way to ensure your herbal garden thrives. In this chapter, we'll explore:

Choosing the Right Location

"Location, location, location!" It's not just real estate agents who harp on this; it's sage advice for your herbal garden too. Not all spaces are created equal, and different herbs have different needs. Are you envisioning an outdoor garden that sprawls under the sun, or a cozy indoor setup next to your kitchen window? We'll help you figure out the best spot for your herbal dreams to take root.

Soil, Sunlight, and Water Needs

Remember, plants are living beings. Just like us, they need a balanced diet and the right living conditions to flourish. We'll dig deep—pun totally intended—into the specifics of soil composition, the sunlight requirements, and just how thirsty your herbs will be. With these elements in harmony, your plants will not only survive but thrive.

Common Herbs and Their Growing Conditions

The stars of the show! Basil, thyme, chamomile—each herb is unique, not just in flavor and medicinal properties but also in how they like to grow. Some are sun-lovers, others prefer the shade. Some like their feet wet, while others prefer to stay dry. Knowing the specific needs of each herb can make the difference between a lush, productive garden and a sad, wilted one. We'll introduce you to some of the most popular and versatile herbs to consider for your garden, along with tips on how to keep them happy and healthy.

By the end of this chapter, you'll be armed with the knowledge you need to set up an herbal garden that not only looks good but also serves your medicinal and culinary needs. It's like putting together a magical puzzle, where each piece—a bit of soil, a splash of water, a ray of sunshine—fits together to create something truly extraordinary: a garden that nourishes both your body and soul. So, roll up your sleeves, put on your gardening gloves, and let's get started!

Choosing the Right Location

Before you get carried away with visions of endless rosemary fields or lavender that wafts into your bedroom window, let's do some reality checks. Not to dampen your enthusiasm, but think of it more as directing your passion towards a garden that will actually grow and flourish.

First things first, take stock of the space you're working with. Do you have a sprawling backyard, a moderate-sized patio, or just a windowsill? The amount of available space significantly influences your choice of location. After all, you wouldn't try to fit a sunflower in a thimble, would you?

And while you're sizing up your space, think about your own lifestyle too. Are you always on the go, or do you have more time to pamper your plants? Your commitment level will also guide the scale and complexity of your garden.

Herbs are a finicky lot when it comes to their love affair with the sun. Some can't get enough of it, bathing themselves in sunlight as if they're at the beach. Others prefer a life in the shade, delicate and reserved. So, how do you strike the right balance?

First off, observe the natural patterns of light and shade in your available space throughout the day. You may notice some areas receive more morning sun, while others are brighter in the afternoon. This intel is gold when planning your garden layout. Sun-loving herbs like rosemary and thyme might enjoy that sunny corner, while shade-loving herbs like mint and parsley would appreciate a spot that's shielded from the afternoon heat.

Soil is not just dirt; it's the lifeblood of your garden. The quality of soil in your chosen location can make or break your herbal dreams. Each herb has its own preference—sandy, loamy, or clayey. While you can amend soil to a certain extent, starting with soil that's already close to your herbs' liking will save you a lot of effort.

A good first step is to get your soil tested. This can give you insights into the soil's pH and nutrient levels, which are crucial for plant health. You might be surprised to find how much your soil's characteristics can vary even within the same yard.

Ever had to deal with waterlogged shoes? It's uncomfortable, right? Well, roots feel the same way about poor drainage. Even moisture-loving herbs don't like to be waterlogged. Make sure your chosen location doesn't become a mini-lake during heavy rain. If it does, consider installing a drainage system or opting for raised beds or containers that you can control more easily.

While we're on the topic of where to plant your herbs, it's worth mentioning that some plants play well together, while others just don't get along. The concept of companion planting goes back centuries and is a fascinating mix of folklore and science. For instance, planting basil next to your tomatoes is said to improve both their health and flavor. However, not every plant is as friendly; some can actually inhibit each other's growth. Doing a bit of research on companion planting can help you maximize your garden's potential.

Your herbs are not just plants; they're a resource. Think about how often you'll need to access them for harvesting or maintenance. The most beautiful garden is not much use if it's a hassle to get to. Keep this in mind when selecting your location. If you use herbs primarily for cooking, having them closer to your kitchen is a wise idea.

Hold up! Before you start tilling and planting, make sure you're aware of any local laws or community guidelines that might affect your gardening plans. In some places, certain plants may be prohibited or require special permits. Also, if you share your space with others, it's respectful to consider how your garden might impact them. Aim to be a good plant parent and a good neighbor.

Last but not least, remember that plants grow—sometimes faster than you'd expect. Make sure to account for the full grown size of the plants, not just their size when you first plant them. Otherwise, you may end up with an overcrowded garden where plants are fighting for space and nutrients.

So there you have it, your in-depth guide to choosing the perfect location for your herbal garden. Remember, the best garden is one that reflects both your needs and the needs of your plants. It's a mutual relationship that, with the right planning, will bring joy and healing for years to come.

So what does your ideal herbal garden look like, and where will it live? Happy pondering and even happier planting!

One often overlooked factor in choosing a location is the concept of 'microclimates.' Every garden, no matter how small, is composed of various microclimates that can influence how well your herbs grow. These are areas where the climate—temperature, moisture, wind, and sunlight—differs from the surrounding zones.

For example, the area by a wall that faces the sun might be perfect for herbs that need more heat and less moisture, as the wall can provide both heat reflection and some protection from rain. Understanding the microclimates in your potential garden space is like unlocking a cheat code for your herbal gardening game.

Seasons change, and so will your garden's conditions. The sunnier spot in the summer could become a frost pocket in winter. Think long-term and understand how the seasons affect your space. Will you need to bring in your potted herbs during winter? Is your area prone to extreme conditions like heavy snow, rainfall, or even drought? Planning for the seasons will ensure that your garden is not just a fleeting summer romance but a long-term commitment.

The choice between planting in the ground and using containers also hinges on your location. Containers are portable and offer more control over soil quality and drainage. They're a great option for patios, balconies, or even indoor spaces. On the other hand, planting in the ground often gives herbs more room to grow and is usually less maintenance-intensive in terms of watering.

Believe it or not, the slight slope in your yard can affect drainage, sunlight, and even the effort you'll need to put into maintaining your garden. Herbs at a higher elevation will generally get more sunlight but may also be exposed to more wind, which can be both a blessing and a curse. A slope can also affect how water drains in your garden, so observe how water flows during a rainy day.

Herbs do more than serve human needs; they're part of a broader ecosystem. Your choice of location could affect the local fauna. Some herbs attract beneficial pollinators like bees and butterflies. At the same time, you might have to consider potential pests. A location that's too isolated may not attract pollinators, while one that's too close to a compost pile or waste area might invite unwanted pests. If you have children or pets, you know they come with their own set of challenges and joys. While the curiosity of a child or a pet can be heartwarming, it can also be disastrous for certain delicate herbs. Some herbs are also not safe for pets or children if ingested. Hence, when selecting a location, ensure it's either out of reach or safe for your household's younger or furrier members.

Finally, it's worth acknowledging the rich traditions that have informed herbal medicine over the centuries. In certain cultures, the location of an herbal garden is chosen with great care, sometimes even involving ritualistic elements. While this may not be everyone's cup of tea (or herbal infusion!), the principle remains: the location of your herbal garden is significant and worth your thoughtful consideration.

So there you have it—more detailed considerations to guide you in choosing the right location for your herbal sanctuary. From understanding your space and climate to considering the needs of both plants and people, there's a lot that goes into this crucial first step of your herbal journey. But remember, it's a labor of love, one that will reward you with not just herbs but a deeper connection to the natural world. Ready to make that dream garden a reality?

For those who turn to herbal remedies as their go-to for minor ailments, having a garden that is both nearby and easily accessible becomes crucial. It's not just about adding flavor to your cooking. You're looking at your basil as a digestive aid or your lavender as a calming force. So, let's take this proximity point a bit further.

How often do you find yourself in need of quick herbal remedies? If you're keen on having a fresh cup of peppermint tea at the first sign of a tummy ache or applying aloe vera straight from the plant for minor burns, then you'll want to place these types of herbs close to your home's entrance or even inside as houseplants. Imagine the convenience of simply stepping outside your kitchen to snip off a piece of aloe or grab some fresh mint leaves.

Now, for those who might have a good amount of space and are looking at a more elaborate garden, zoning becomes essential. In permaculture, zoning is a design method that places elements according to how often you need to access them. Herbs you use daily, like basil or mint, should be in Zone 1, closest to your house. Those that require less frequent attention can be placed further away in Zone 2 or even Zone 3.

While this might sound like a leap into the esoteric, there are age-old traditions that speak to the idea that the energy flow within a space can affect living things, plants included. Feng Shui, an ancient Chinese practice, believes in harmonizing everyone with their surrounding environment. For the skeptics out there, it might be a little 'out there,' but why not experiment a little? Try positioning your herbs in a manner that aligns with Feng Shui principles and see if it makes a difference in your garden's harmony and productivity. At the very least, it will make for a fun gardening experiment.

Who said gardens have to be horizontal? When space is at a premium, or even just for aesthetic pleasure, considering vertical options can be a game-changer. Wall-mounted planters, hanging baskets, or even custom-built vertical plant walls can offer a unique twist to your herbal garden. However, remember that elevation can also mean increased exposure to elements like wind, so choose hardy herbs for these elevated spots.

Did you know that some herbs prefer cold weather, while others need the heat to truly thrive? Cilantro, for example, is a cool-season herb. It might not survive the height of summer but would happily grow in the fall or spring. On the other hand, basil loves the heat. By understanding the seasonal preferences of your herbs, you could keep your garden productive all year round. Your chosen location should then allow for this flexibility, perhaps with space for portable pots that can be moved in or out depending on the season.

There's history in the soil. What was your garden before it became your 'garden'? Was it a flowerbed, a dumping ground, or maybe even another herb garden? Knowing the area's previous use can provide insights into soil quality and what kinds of plants it can support. If it was an herb garden before, you might find that some herbs naturally flourish in this space, thanks to years of soil enrichment.

Lastly, but certainly not least, consider the aesthetic aspect. While the primary purpose of your herbal garden is functional—to provide herbs—it's also a part of your home. The visual appeal of the garden can add to your overall well-being. You'll be more motivated to spend time in a space that is not just productive but also beautiful. Arrange herbs with varying heights and colors together. Add pathways, pebbles, or even fairy lights. The sky's the limit, really!

Picking the perfect location for your herbal garden is like setting the stage for a grand performance. The better the stage, the more magnificent the performance. Your herbs, those little bursts of aroma and flavor, are the stars. Your commitment, research, and thoughtful planning are the directors of this show. Once the stage is set right, you're in for an aromatic, therapeutic, and absolutely magical journey. So, what's stopping you? Ready to roll up those sleeves and start plotting your herbal paradise?

Soil, Sunlight, and Water Needs

Think of soil as a mini-universe bustling with life. Sure, it's made up of minerals like sand, silt, and clay, but it also houses a community of microscopic organisms—bacteria, fungi, and even tiny insects. Each contributes to the soil's health and, consequently, the well-being of your plants. Soil is not just 'dirt'; it's an ecosystem.

Just like humans, different herbs prefer different types of soil. While most culinary herbs prefer well-drained, loamy soil, some herbs, like mint and chives, are quite forgiving and will grow in a variety of soil types. But then there are finicky ones, like lavender, which prefer sandy soil that mimics their Mediterranean origin.

Soil pH can make or break your garden. Most herbs prefer a neutral to slightly acidic soil pH range of 6.0 to 7.0. However, there are exceptions. For example, rosemary and thyme prefer a more alkaline soil. Testing your soil's pH is not just for the geeks; it's for anyone who wants a thriving garden. Nowadays, you can easily find soil testing kits online or at your local garden store.

The excitement of planting often overshadows soil preparation, but this step is crucial. Depending on what was previously grown in your chosen location, you might need to remove weeds, rocks, and other debris. Incorporating organic matter like compost enriches the soil and improves its texture and drainage. Trust me, your future herbs will thank you for this.

Not all soil issues are visible to the naked eye. Sometimes, problems like soil compaction can lurk beneath the surface. Compacted soil can restrict root growth and water absorption. Before planting, it's advisable to dig a few test holes to check the soil's deeper layers. If it feels too hard, it might need some amending, usually by adding organic matter and aerating the soil.

Now, let's pivot to something equally crucial but perhaps more visible: Sunlight.

You might think light is light. Well, plants would respectfully disagree. Sunlight contains a spectrum of colors, each with its own wavelength. Blue light helps with plant growth, while red light aids in flowering. When picking a location for your garden, consider not just the amount of light but also the quality of it.

Herbs like basil, oregano, and rosemary love the sun and need at least 6-8 hours of it each day. But then you have herbs like mint and parsley that prefer partial shade. You'll need to consider these individual requirements when planning your garden. And it's not just about what these plants want but also about what they can tolerate. For instance, cilantro will bolt (produce flowers and seeds) quickly in hot, sunny conditions, essentially ending its lifecycle prematurely.

Sunlight is not just about duration but also timing. Morning sunlight is generally considered gentler and less drying compared to the harsh afternoon sun. Herbs like chervil and dill that prefer partial shade would appreciate a spot that gets morning sun and afternoon shade.

The sun doesn't remain constant throughout the year; it takes different paths across the sky. This can drastically affect how much sunlight your garden receives. Some areas may be sunny in the summer but shady in the winter. It's crucial to consider these seasonal shifts when choosing your garden's location.

Speaking of water—let's dive right into it.

While we're used to just turning on the tap to water our gardens, have you ever stopped to consider the quality of the water you're using? Tap water often contains chlorine, which is not exactly plant-friendly. Rainwater is the gold standard when it comes to watering your herbs. If possible, consider setting up a rainwater harvesting system. Not only is it better for your plants, but it's also more sustainable.

Drip, Sprinkle, or Soak?

Different herbs have different water requirements. Mediterranean herbs like lavender, rosemary, and oregano are used to dry conditions and prefer less frequent, more deep watering. In contrast, herbs like basil and mint prefer the soil to be consistently moist. Understanding these needs will guide you in choosing the right watering technique, whether it's a traditional watering can, a hose, or a more advanced drip irrigation system.

Evaporation is a constant enemy for gardeners, especially during the hot summer months. One of the best ways to combat this is by applying a layer of mulch around your plants. Mulch not only helps retain moisture but also improves soil quality and inhibits weed growth.

Too much of a good thing can be bad, and that applies to water as well. Herbs generally don't like to sit in waterlogged soil. Good drainage is essential, and that's another reason why soil preparation is crucial. Raised beds or planting in pots can also help improve drainage.

While we're on the subject of water, let's talk timing. You might think, "Hey, as long as the plants are getting water, we're good, right?" Well, not quite. Watering in the early morning or late afternoon minimizes evaporation, making your watering more efficient. Also, water droplets on leaves can act like tiny magnifying glasses, focusing sunlight and potentially causing leaf burn. So, it's better to water when the sun is low.

We touched on drainage earlier, but let's delve deeper. Too much water can lead to root rot, a fatal condition for most herbs. If you find that your garden's soil is retaining too much water, you might need to incorporate more sand or organic matter to improve drainage. In extreme cases, you might even consider installing a French drain system.

Don't discount the role of natural rainfall in your watering schedule. If it's been a particularly rainy week, adjust your watering schedule accordingly. Some smart irrigation systems can even sync with weather forecasts to automate this for you.

Now that we've showered you with insights on water let's switch gears and look at something just as fluid but less tangible: climate and microclimates.

Understanding Your Garden's Microclimate

What's a Microclimate Anyway?

So you've probably heard of climate zones, those large swathes of land that share similar weather patterns. But let's zoom in. Microclimates are localized climate conditions that can differ significantly from the general climate of an area. Think of that sunny spot next to your fence where snow seems to melt first, or that perpetually shady corner under the tree.

Why should you care? Well, understanding the microclimates in your garden can help you position your herbs for maximum success. That sun-loving rosemary might thrive next to the south-facing wall, while your shade-loving mint might be happiest under the dappled shade of a tree.

And guess what? You can even create your own microclimates! Planting windbreaks, installing shade cloths, or creating raised beds can all alter your garden's local climate, tailoring it to better meet your herbs' needs.

Seasonal Considerations: Your Garden Through the Year

If you're gardening in a region with frosty winters, this part is for you. Some herbs are perennial, meaning they'll come back year after year. Others, like basil, are annuals and won't survive frost. Knowing the first and last frost dates for your area can guide your planting schedule.

Planting only in spring is so last century! Seasonal succession planting lets you have a vibrant garden throughout the year. After your summer basil has bolted, why not plant some fall-loving cilantro or winter-hardy chives?

Alright, friends, there's a ton more we could dive into, like troubleshooting common garden issues or planning for pollinators, but alas, let's take a breather for now. I hope you're feeling more empowered and excited to embark on your herbal gardening journey! Your garden is more than just a plot of land; it's a living, breathing ecosystem, and you're the steward. So, are you ready to step into your new role?

We've covered a lot of ground, so to speak, and hopefully provided you with the foundational knowledge to cultivate a flourishing herbal garden. And remember, your journey into herbalism is just like planting a seed—you may not see results overnight, but with care and patience, beautiful things will grow.

So, are you ready to get your hands dirty? I can't wait to hear about your herbal adventures!

Common Herbs and Their Growing Conditions

Herbs are the spice of the gardening world. From culinary favorites like basil and oregano to medicinal workhorses like echinacea and peppermint, the variety is staggering. Each of these plant characters has its own back story, unique needs, and special talents. So let's roll up our sleeves and meet some of them, shall we?

Basil: The Summer Superstar

Let's start with a crowd-pleaser, shall we? Basil is the cool kid in the herb world. If your garden was a high school, basil would be the prom king or queen—popular, versatile, and easy to get along with. Basil loves sun and warm temperatures, making it an ideal summer crop. This herb thrives in well-drained, nutrient-rich soil. But here's a pro tip: don't get too eager and plant it before the last frost. Basil is sensitive to cold and will turn black at the slightest chill.

Rosemary: The Hardy Pioneer

On the flip side, we have rosemary, a rugged herb that almost relishes neglect. Originating from the Mediterranean, this herb is used to hot, dry conditions. It prefers well-drained soil, and overwatering is a common mistake. Rosemary can be a perennial in zones 7-10, meaning it could be your garden's loyal friend year after year. But wait, there's a twist! Rosemary is not just a one-trick pony; different varieties like 'Arp' and 'Madeline Hill' have been developed for colder climates.

Lavender: The Fragrant Diva

Now let's talk about lavender, the diva of the herb world. This herb not only brings its aromatic beauty to your garden but also serves multiple purposes, from culinary to medicinal and even ornamental. Like rosemary, it hails from the Mediterranean and prefers well-drained soil and lots of sunlight. Lavender, however, is a bit fussy about its soil. It likes it slightly alkaline, so you may need to amend your soil with lime to hit that sweet spot.

Mint: The Unstoppable Force

Let's switch gears to mint, the herb that could probably grow on a rock if given a chance. It's invasive, spreading through runners, so consider planting it in containers unless you want a minty lawn. This herb loves moist soil and can tolerate partial shade. But beware, mint is like that friend who overstays their welcome; if you don't set boundaries (or in this case, barriers), it will take over your garden.

Thyme: The Understated Workhorse

Thyme is one of those herbs that quietly does its job without demanding much attention. This low-growing perennial loves full sun but will tolerate partial shade. It's drought-resistant and prefers well-drained soil. The many varieties offer a range of flavors and fragrances—from lemon thyme to caraway thyme.

Chamomile: The Night-Time Charmer

Alright, let's talk about chamomile, the darling of bedtime teas. This daisy-like herb is not only a beauty to behold but also has a plethora of medicinal uses. Guess what? It's pretty forgiving when it comes to soil quality. Although it prefers well-drained soil, it can tolerate some pretty poor conditions too. As for sunlight, chamomile is one of those laid-back friends who's happy in full sun but doesn't mind a little afternoon shade.

Cilantro: The Love-It-or-Hate-It Herb

Cilantro! Some people love it; others think it tastes like soap. But we're not here to debate taste buds. When it comes to growing conditions, cilantro is pretty low-maintenance. It likes well-drained soil and prefers full sun, although it can tolerate some shade. A quick heads up: cilantro has a short life and tends to bolt (that is, flower and go to seed) quickly, especially in hot conditions. So it's a good idea to sow a new batch every few weeks if you want a continuous supply.

Sage: The Herb of Wisdom

They say sage is for wisdom, and you'll certainly be wise to include it in your herbal garden. This perennial herb is pretty low-maintenance and thrives in well-drained, sandy, loamy soil. It's drought-tolerant once established and prefers full sun. Sage is also quite hardy and can survive colder temperatures, making it a great option for various climates.

Parsley: The Underestimated Garnish

Let's not forget parsley, often sidelined as just a garnish but offering so much more. This herb loves rich, moist soil and will tolerate either full sun or partial shade. Here's a little secret: parsley is a biennial plant, meaning it'll stick around for two years. The first year is all about the leaves, but it'll produce flowers and seeds in its second year. Once it seeds, however, the leaves can become bitter, so you may want to plant a new batch each year for culinary use.

Oregano: The Pizza's Best Friend

Last but not least in this round-up, let's talk about oregano. This perennial herb is a staple in Italian and Greek cuisine and offers a burst of flavor with its aromatic leaves. Oregano is incredibly forgiving, thriving in just about any soil type as long as it has good drainage. This herb loves basking in full sun and is drought-tolerant once established.

Dill: The Butterfly Attractor

Moving on, let's talk about dill, the herb that's as good in pickles as it is at attracting butterflies to your garden. It's an annual herb, which means you'll have to plant it anew each season, but the delightful yellow flowers and feathery leaves are totally worth it. Dill likes a sunny spot but can tolerate a little bit of shade. And talk about being low-maintenance; it's drought-resistant and thrives in well-drained, slightly acidic to neutral soil.

Echinacea: The Immunity Booster

Echinacea, popularly known as the purple coneflower, is a must-have if you're into medicinal herbs. Not only are the flowers stunning, but they're also potent immunity boosters. This perennial prefers well-drained soil and thrives in full sun. You'll find echinacea to be pretty drought-resistant once established. Plus, it attracts pollinators like bees and butterflies, making it a garden superstar.

Fennel: The Licorice Impersonator

Fennel! With its feathery leaves and licorice-like flavor, it's a versatile herb that deserves a spot in your garden. Be mindful, though; fennel can be somewhat invasive, so it might be wise to plant it where it can spread without causing havoc among its plant neighbors. This herb loves full sun and can tolerate a range of soil types, although it prefers slightly acidic conditions.

Lemon Balm: The Stress Reliever

Now, how about a herb that smells like lemon and helps relieve stress? Enter lemon balm. This herb is a member of the mint family and shares some of the same easy-to-grow attributes. Lemon balm thrives in full sun to partial shade and prefers well-drained, sandy, loamy soil. It's perennial in zones 4-9, so chances are you'll have it as a garden companion for years.

Nasturtium: The Edible Ornament

Last but not least, let's talk about nasturtiums. These aren't just pretty faces; both their flowers and leaves are edible. They have a peppery kick and make a colorful addition to salads. Nasturtiums are super easy to grow, thriving in poor, well-drained soil and full sun to partial shade. If your soil is too rich, you'll get lush leaves but few flowers, so go easy on the fertilizer.

Ginger: The Tropical Delight

Okay, let's switch gears a bit and talk about ginger. This tropical native isn't what you'd typically expect in a North American or European garden, but it's incredibly rewarding to grow. You start with the rhizomes—those knobbly bits you're used to seeing in grocery stores. Plant them in rich, well-drained soil, but here's the kicker: ginger loves humidity and warmth. This might be an indoor project if you're living somewhere cooler, or perhaps a greenhouse endeavor.

Horseradish: The Spicy Outlier

Last but not least for this round is horseradish, a root herb that packs a spicy punch. It prefers full sun but can tolerate partial shade and isn't too picky about soil types. But be warned: like mint, horseradish can become invasive. Once it gets going, it really gets going, so consider planting it in a designated area or in a large pot.

Chapter 3: Essential Tools for the Herbalist

As you venture deeper into the fascinating world of herbal medicine and gardening, you'll soon realize that your hands and intuition, though indispensable, won't be the only tools you'll need.

In this chapter, we'll walk you through the foundational gear and techniques that'll make your herbal journey not only easier but also safer and more rewarding. Just like a painter needs brushes and a canvas, or a musician needs an instrument and a tune, you'll need some basic equipment and guidelines to bring your herbal visions to life.

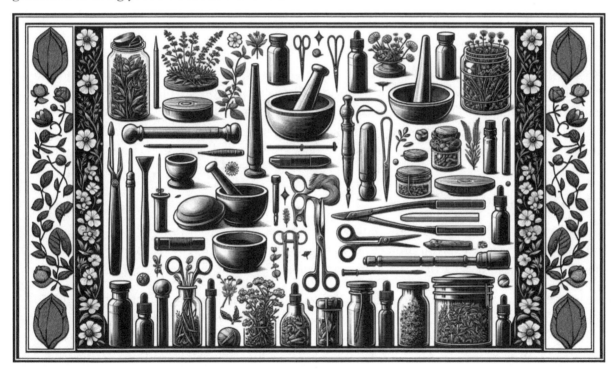

What's Ahead?

Basic Tools and Equipment: From trowels for digging to jars for storing your concoctions, we'll give you the lowdown on all the must-have tools that will make you a better herbalist. You wouldn't embark on a road trip without a map and a well-stocked car, right? Similarly, getting the right tools is crucial for ensuring a successful and joyful herbal journey.

Safety Protocols in Handling and Storage: Being a responsible herbalist means not just taking care of plants but also taking care of yourself and others. The herbs we love can offer incredible benefits, but they also come with their own sets of precautions. You'll need to know how to handle them safely and store them in a way that preserves their potency while minimizing risks. It's not just about doing things right; it's about doing the right things, safely.

So put on your metaphorical (or literal!) gardening gloves, and let's dive into the essential toolkit of the modern herbalist. Trust me, you're going to relish this part of the journey; it's where things get tactile and exciting. After all, who doesn't love acquiring a few nifty gadgets to enhance their favorite hobby? Especially when that hobby brings well-being to you and those you care about.

Ready? Let's venture forth!

Basic Tools and Equipment

Rakes, Hoes, and Garden Forks

Earlier, we chatted about trowels and gloves, but what about the other heroes of the herb garden? A rake isn't just a prop in horror movies; it's a valuable asset when you want to smooth soil or gather up debris like leaves or cuttings. The type of rake you'll need depends on your garden's layout and size. A flathead rake works well for leveling and smoothing soil, while a leaf rake comes in handy for cleaning up leaves and other light debris.

Hoes and garden forks also deserve their moment in the spotlight. Hoes are perfect for breaking up hard soil and weeding between your beloved plants. Garden forks, on the other hand, are better for digging and aerating soil. There are different types of hoes and forks—each designed for specific tasks. A Dutch hoe, for instance, is excellent for weeding, while a pronged garden fork is ideal for turning compost. When selecting these tools, consider ergonomic designs to minimize strain on your back and hands.

Trowels, Gloves, and Shears

Let's start where all good herbs do: the garden. Your hands will be your primary tool here, but a good pair of gloves will help you protect them. Digging in the earth is soul-satisfying, but your hands will thank you for a barrier against blisters, calluses, and dirt.

Next in line are trowels and gardening shears. Trowels are essential for transplanting herbs and digging small holes for seeds. Choose one with a sturdy, comfortable handle, as you'll be using this tool frequently. Gardening shears are your go-to for snipping herbs in a way that encourages new growth and maintains the plant's health. Look for shears with a safety lock and rust-resistant blades. If you have roses among your herbs for making rose water or rosehip oil, consider specialized pruning shears.

Mortar and Pestle, Mesh Strainers, and Funnels

The preparation of herbs often requires that they be crushed or ground to release their oils and essences. For this, a mortar and pestle set is your best friend. They come in various materials such as porcelain, stone, and wood. Each type has its pros and cons, but for a good all-rounder, consider a granite set. Its rough texture is great for grinding both dry and wet ingredients.

Mesh strainers and funnels are less glamorous but crucial. You'll be using strainers for filtering herbal infusions, tinctures, and oils. A stainless steel mesh is a good choice for its durability and ease of cleaning. As for funnels, they are lifesavers when you're transferring your freshly made liquid gold—be it essential oils, tinctures, or balms—into storage bottles.

Glass Jars, Labels, and Dropper Bottles

You've put in all the hard work growing, harvesting, and preparing your herbs, so how you store them is of utmost importance. Glass jars with airtight lids are indispensable for storing dried herbs, tinctures, and oils. Clear jars are fine for items you'll store in dark cupboards, but for light-sensitive preparations, amber or cobalt blue jars are ideal. Labels are equally crucial; you don't want to mix up your chamomile and valerian root, especially not at bedtime! Invest in waterproof, smudge-proof labels.

Dropper bottles are fantastic for storing essential oils and tinctures. They allow you to dispense your herbal products drop by drop, minimizing waste and making it easy to administer precise doses.

Scales, Measuring Cups, and Notebooks

Precision matters in herbalism. Digital scales are essential for weighing herbs and other ingredients. This is especially true when you're following a recipe or making a product where dosage is crucial, like medicinal tinctures. Measuring cups and spoons are basics you probably already have in your kitchen, but consider getting a set just for herbal preparations to avoid cross-contamination with food ingredients.

Last but not least, a good old-fashioned notebook—or a digital one if you're more the typing sort. Keeping records of what you plant, when you harvest, and how you prepare your herbal products is invaluable. Your notebook becomes a personalized guide and a record of your herbal journey.

Gloves and Masks

Not all herbs are friendly; some can irritate your skin or produce strong fumes. A pair of nitrile gloves can offer good protection during preparation and handling. When you're working with particularly potent herbs or essential oils, you may also want to consider a face mask to protect against inhaling any irritants.

Dehydrators and Oil Press Machines

While not strictly "basic," these modern devices can simplify and streamline some of the more time-consuming aspects of herbalism. A dehydrator can significantly speed up the drying process for your herbs, ensuring they retain maximum potency. An oil press machine can be a worthwhile investment if you're planning to make large quantities of herbal oils.

Planters, Drip Trays, and Grow Lights

If you don't have the luxury of outdoor space or if you're dealing with unforgiving winters, indoor herb gardening can be a great alternative. Here, planters become your soil and universe. There are many types of planters: ceramic, terracotta, plastic, or even fabric ones like grow bags. Each has its pros and cons. For example, ceramic pots are porous and allow the soil to breathe but can be heavy and breakable. Plastic pots are lightweight and durable but may not offer great drainage.

Drip trays save your indoor surfaces from water damage, and many come with planters as a set. However, make sure to empty the drip tray regularly to avoid root rot from stagnant water.

Grow lights can be a lifesaver during those gloomy months when natural light is scarce. LED grow lights have become quite affordable and are energy-efficient. They can offer a full spectrum of light, simulating natural sunlight for your indoor herbs. If you're venturing into indoor growing, invest in timers for your grow lights to replicate a natural day-night cycle.

Double Boilers, Thermometers, and PH Meters

In the realm of preparation, there's another layer of complexity we haven't touched on: heat and acidity. Some herbal concoctions, like salves and certain tinctures, require precise temperatures. A double boiler provides a gentle, even heat—perfect for melting beeswax or simmering herbal infusions. Add a candy or meat thermometer to your toolkit to monitor temperatures accurately.

While we're talking about measurements, let's not overlook the pH meter. Certain herbs, particularly those used for medicinal teas or tinctures, have specific pH requirements. A digital pH meter can help you ensure that your preparations meet these requirements, which is vital for both safety and effectiveness.

The Herbalist's Library 2.0: Apps and Software

Though a physical notebook has a rustic appeal, don't dismiss the convenience of digital note-keeping. There are numerous apps and software designed for gardeners and herbalists. These digital platforms can offer features like photo logging, weather tracking, and even plant identification using AI. The advantage of digital note-keeping is the ability to search and update your logs easily.

Large Containers and Vacuum Sealers

If you're planning to go all-in and prepare herbs on a grand scale, your storage needs will also scale up. Large, food-grade plastic or stainless steel containers can be invaluable for storing large quantities of dried herbs or liquid preparations like oils and tinctures. Vacuum sealers can further extend the shelf life of dried herbs by removing air from the packaging, slowing down the oxidation process.

Aprons, Hand Creams, and First-Aid Kits

A few final additions that might not immediately come to mind but can be essential are a sturdy apron, a good hand cream, and a basic first-aid kit. An apron with pockets can keep your smaller tools and even your notebook within easy reach. Gardening and handling herbs can dry out your skin, so a good hand cream can be a lifesaver. And a first-aid kit is always good to have around, just in case of minor cuts or insect bites.

Now that we've thoroughly explored the nooks and crannies of a well-stocked herbalist's toolkit, you should feel well-prepared to handle nearly any task that comes your way. What seemed overwhelming at first is now an exciting shopping list, each item a stepping stone on your herbal journey. The key takeaway? Equip yourself wisely, and your herbal endeavors will be more efficient, more effective, and, most importantly, more enjoyable. So, what are you waiting for? Your herbalist's toolkit is a realm waiting to be populated!

By now, your virtual shopping cart might be full, but remember, you don't have to get everything at once. Start with the essentials that align most closely with your immediate interests, and build up your toolkit over time. Just like your garden, your collection of tools will grow as you do, branching out in new directions with each season of your herbal journey.

Armed with the right tools, your path into herbalism will be that much smoother and more enjoyable. So, what are you most excited about adding to your toolkit?

Safety Protocols in Handling and Storage

While it's easy to get swept up in the excitement of your newfound herbal journey, it's equally important to take a step back and consider the safety aspects. Safety, after all, is like the seatbelt of herbalism—it's what ensures that your voyage through the fascinating world of plants is smooth and hazard-free.

First things first, let's talk about safe handling, which actually starts way before the herbs have even been picked. Think about it: if you're sourcing herbs from a public area or even your own backyard, it's crucial to know if those areas have been exposed to pesticides, fungicides, or other chemical treatments. Even a beautifully vibrant looking plant can harbor harmful substances if grown in contaminated soil. That's why it's essential to either grow your herbs organically or source them from trusted places that can verify their purity.

Handling the herbs properly extends to the tools you use. Remember the pair of garden shears we talked about? They shouldn't just be sharp; they should also be clean. And not just swipe-with-a-tissue clean, but sanitized using rubbing alcohol or hydrogen peroxide. The same goes for other tools you might use for cutting, grinding, or mashing herbs. Bacteria and mold spores are always lurking about, eager to hitch a ride on your freshly harvested lavender or mint. Keeping your tools clean helps ensure that your herbal preparations remain pure and beneficial.

Gloves can be your best friend, especially when dealing with herbs that have irritants or strong natural dyes. Plants like stinging nettle or turmeric can leave their mark, either through a rash or a stubborn stain. So, it's wise to don a pair of gloves when handling these, even if you think you have the steady hands of a surgeon. If you think this is taking it a step too far, just consider it a barrier between you and potential skin irritation or allergies, especially when handling plants like poison ivy or even some types of mushrooms that could be growing in your herb garden.

Once you've harvested or obtained your herbs, the next step is usually drying them. Now, a well-ventilated area is key for this. If moisture lingers, it creates an environment that's conducive to the growth of mold. So, while it might be tempting to hang your rosemary sprigs in a cute little bundle above the fireplace, that's often not the best option unless you're sure that the area has good air circulation and is free from moisture. Investing in a good-quality dehumidifier can often save you a lot of heartache, not to mention ruined herbs.

Now, on to storage, the chapter of our safety story where the stakes get even higher. We've all seen those apothecary jars filled with vibrant-colored herbs. They look beautiful, yes, but glass jars aren't just about aesthetics. Glass doesn't react with the herbs, meaning it won't compromise the quality of what's stored inside. However, the lid also matters. It should be airtight, and if possible, the glass should be tinted to protect the herbs from light degradation. If tinted jars aren't an option, storing them in a dark cabinet can do the trick. Just make sure it's a cool and dry environment.

Don't forget to label your jars. It sounds simple, but you'd be surprised how similar dried basil and dried oregano can look after a few weeks on the shelf. And let's not even get into the confusion that can occur with powdered roots and barks. Labeling can save you from culinary mishaps and medicinal mix-ups. Mention the herb, the date of storage, and any other relevant details like whether it's the root, leaf, or flower that's stored.

Temperature is another factor. While a cool, dark cupboard is generally a safe bet, certain preparations like infused oils might need to be stored in a refrigerator, especially if they're made with fresh herbs. Humidity and temperature can affect the oil's shelf life and can even lead to spoilage.

Let's take a moment to talk about kids and pets. They're curious creatures and will almost certainly be drawn to your collection of herbs and herbal preparations. Childproof caps on bottles and a dedicated cupboard with a lock can make all the difference in keeping both your stash and your family safe. This applies to herbs that are toxic or have strong effects but extends to all herbs for good measure.

While safety often revolves around prevention, it's also about informed usage. This means knowing the dosage, interactions, and side effects of the herbs you're using, particularly for internal consumption. You don't need to go to medical school to be a responsible herbalist, but a good guidebook or trusted online resources can go a long way. Knowing the difference between a therapeutic and a toxic dose is crucial. Same goes for potential interactions with medications you might already be taking.

Herbalism, as a practice, has thrived for thousands of years because our ancestors knew the importance of treating plants with respect. This reverence for the natural world goes hand in hand with understanding its limitations and potential for harm. And that's where safety protocols are rooted—in knowledge and respect. So, as you continue on your herbal journey, keep these safety guidelines in mind. They're not just rules but pathways that guide you toward a more fulfilling and safe exploration of the herbal world. Your practice can only be enriched by the careful attention you give to the seemingly mundane details of safety. And remember, a well-prepared herbalist is not just a wise herbalist but also a safe one.

Preparation, where the magic happens! It's where you channel your inner alchemist to transform simple plants into balms, tinctures, oils, and teas. But remember, even alchemists of yore were particular about their protocols. One wrong move, and you're not turning lead into gold—you're turning a helpful herb into a harmful one.

Take essential oils, for example. These potent elixirs are concentrated forms of the plant's beneficial properties. But their potency can also mean toxicity at higher doses. A drop too many of, say, clove oil, and you can go from curing a toothache to suffering from burns in your mouth. This is where dilution comes in. Essential oils, with few exceptions, should be diluted in a carrier oil before application. Grapeseed oil, jojoba oil, or even olive oil can serve as good carriers, offering a buffer that allows you to safely harness the benefits of the essential oil.

The same logic applies to tinctures. These alcohol-based extracts can last for years and are an excellent way to preserve the medicinal properties of herbs. However, a common mistake many new herbalists make is confusing the dosage of a tincture with that of a tea. Remember, tinctures are concentrated. One dropper can be equivalent to an entire cup of herbal tea. So, when you're following a recipe or a guide, pay close attention to the recommended dosage, and err on the side of caution. It's always easier to take a little more later than to deal with the consequences of taking too much.

And speaking of sharing, isn't that one of the joys of diving into the world of herbal medicine? You discover a fantastic remedy and you just have to let your friends and family in on it. But here's where you need to tread lightly. What works for you may not work for everyone. Allergies, current medications, and existing health conditions can turn an otherwise benign herb into a potential hazard. Always recommend that they consult a healthcare provider, especially for serious conditions or if they're already on medication. Just like you wouldn't want someone prescribing you medicine willy-nilly, you should exercise the same caution when recommending herbal remedies to others.

Another layer of complexity arises when we consider the changing nature of herbs themselves. Plants are not static beings; they're influenced by soil quality, weather conditions, and even the time of day when they're harvested. This means the potency of an herb can vary from one batch to another. So, even if you've used it successfully before, it's good to start with lower doses and work your way up, just to account for any natural variances in potency.

A special word for those adventurous souls who like to wildcraft their herbs—that is, gather them from the great outdoors. While it can be incredibly rewarding to forage for your own herbs, this practice comes with its own set of safety concerns. Accurate identification is paramount. A simple mistake can mean the difference between picking a healing herb and a toxic one. Always double or even triple-check using reputable field guides or, better yet, the expertise of seasoned foragers.

We often think of herbalism as a solitary practice, a communion between you and the plant world. But there's also a community aspect to it. A seasoned herbalist will tell you that one of their most valued resources is their network of fellow herbalists. This network can be a treasure trove of shared knowledge, advice, and, most importantly, safety tips. So, engage with communities, whether online or in person. Attend workshops, webinars, and herb walks. The collective wisdom you'll gain is invaluable not only for expanding your expertise but also for honing your safety protocols.

In conclusion, the world of herbalism is as vast as it is ancient. Its roots stretch back through centuries, woven into the very fabric of human history. But while the herbs have remained the same, our understanding of them continues to evolve. By coupling ancient wisdom with modern safety practices, you're not just honoring the tradition of herbalism—you're actively contributing to its evolution. The herbs give us their gifts abundantly; let's do them the honor of using these gifts wisely and safely. It's not just about preventing harm but also about maximizing benefit, for yourself and for all those you share your herbal wisdom with.

So, as you embark further on your herbal journey, may your steps be as sure as they are curious, your methods as careful as they are creative. This is how you become not just an herbalist, but a guardian of an ancient, living tradition. Happy herbing!

Chapter 4: Crafting Essential Oils

Welcome to Chapter 4, where we dive into the alchemy of these concentrated liquid gems. They're like your favorite herbs and flowers, but distilled down to their very essence, each drop a microcosm of botanical power. Imagine walking through a lavender field, the air almost palpable with scent. Essential oils are like bottling up that experience to revisit whenever you please.

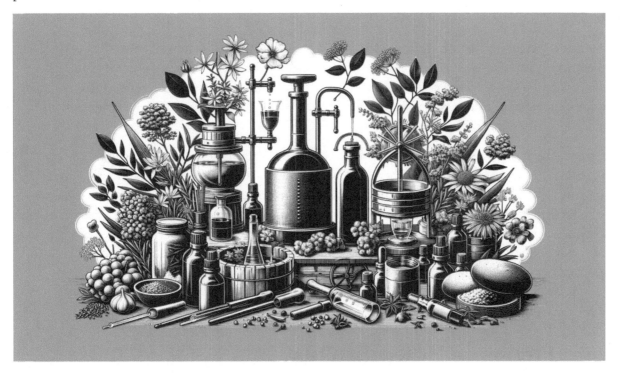

But let's demystify them a bit. Essential oils aren't just pretty fragrances; they're the lifeblood of plants, packed with compounds that give each plant its unique characteristics, from the lavender's calming vibes to peppermint's invigorating zing. And we're not the first generation to be smitten with these oils. Oh no, our ancestors from various cultures were ahead of us, using rudimentary distillation techniques to extract oils for rituals, medicines, and, yes, even for cosmetics. So, when you're dabbling with essential oils, you're part of a lineage that spans both time and geography.

However, while our ancestors may have been limited by the technology of their times, we certainly aren't. The ways in which we can extract essential oils have evolved, becoming both more efficient and eco-friendly. Steam distillation is currently the reigning champ. Imagine a sauna but for plants, where steam helps release the oil, which is then condensed back into a liquid. Then, of course, there's cold pressing, often used for citrus oils. Imagine squeezing an orange peel so hard that the oils burst forth—that's cold pressing in a nutshell, or should I say, a peel?

For those of you who fancy a bit of a science experiment, solvent extraction is another option, although it's usually reserved for fragile flowers like jasmine that might not survive the intensity of steam. However, it's crucial to remember that you're working with potent solvents, so let's not get too carried away playing mad scientist, okay?

Let's face it; these extraction methods sound like something out of a Hogwarts Potions class. And just like potions, essential oils require a certain level of respect and care. We've already discussed how potent they are. Well, with great power comes great responsibility—yes, even Spider-Man would agree! So, after you've successfully extracted your oils or bought a high-quality bottle, where do you keep it? A cool, dark place is your best bet. Trust me, you don't want to expose these oils to heat, light, or oxygen if you can avoid it. That's like leaving a chocolate bar in the sun—a waste of something good. And, oh, please do invest in dark-colored glass bottles. Your oils will thank you for the TLC.

While we're on the subject of tender loving care, let's not forget our own well-being. Safety first, remember? Just because essential oils are natural doesn't make them universally safe. Dilute before applying, do a patch test, and consult a healthcare provider if you're pregnant, nursing, or managing any chronic health conditions. It's also a good idea to be aware of potential interactions with any medications you're on.

So, from their humble plant origins to the wizardry of extraction methods, essential oils are a fascinating journey into the heart of herbalism. They invite us to explore, to experiment, and to experience the natural world in one of its most potent forms. But they also remind us that nature is not to be trifled with; respect for these oils and the plants they come from is the cornerstone of safe and effective use. And that, my friends, is the beauty and the wisdom of essential oils. They link us to the world around us, asking us to slow down, to pay attention, and to honor the natural abundance that so generously enriches our lives. Happy crafting!

Introduction to Essential Oils

What is it about these tiny bottles that so captures our imagination? Is it the allure of the exotic scents—jasmine from India, sandalwood from Australia? Or maybe it's the promise of transformative health benefits, those whispers of easing stress, boosting immunity, or even enhancing spirituality? In this section, we'll delve into what makes essential oils such a cornerstone in both traditional and contemporary practices of herbal medicine, and why they might just deserve a space on your shelf.

Imagine strolling through a lavender field on a sunny day, the purple blooms swaying gently in the wind, butterflies and bees busy at work, and that heavenly scent filling the air. Now, imagine capturing the essence of that experience in a tiny glass bottle you can take anywhere. That's what essential oils offer—a concentrated experience of nature, made possible through a fascinating blend of tradition and technology. These oils are literally the "essence" of the plant, containing its aroma and therapeutic properties, neatly packed into a potent liquid form.

But don't let their modern packaging fool you. Essential oils have a rich history dating back thousands of years. Whether it was the ancient Egyptians incorporating them in their embalming practices or the medieval Europeans using them to ward off plague (they thought it was effective, at least), these oils have played an integral role in various civilizations. Hippocrates, the Father of Medicine, is said to have practiced aromatherapy with fennel, and even prescribed it for digestive issues. And if we venture eastward, we'll find that Ayurveda, the ancient Indian system of medicine, has long been singing the praises of oils like sandalwood and eucalyptus.

While history provides a compelling backstory, let's not forget the role essential oils play in the modern world. With the resurgence of holistic health and wellness trends, essential oils are enjoying a sort of renaissance. They're no longer confined to the cabinets of your grandma who swears by her tea tree oil for every malady, or that one hippie friend who dabs patchouli oil like it's going out of style. No, essential oils have entered the mainstream, finding their way into everything from high-end skincare products to everyday household cleaners.

Now, you might be asking, "How do we get from plant to bottle?" That's where the art of extraction comes in. There's a certain alchemy involved, and it feels almost magical. Traditional methods like steam distillation are still prevalent. Imagine a giant kettle filled with aromatic herbs. Steam rises through the plant material, liberating the oils, which are then cooled down to form a liquid. It's like brewing a very intense cup of herbal tea, only a lot more potent. But we also have modern methods, like supercritical CO_2 extraction, which use carbon dioxide to obtain lighter and more delicate oils. This is particularly useful for extracting oils from delicate flowers like jasmine or neroli, which might otherwise lose their aroma in the steaming process.

So far, so good, right? But once you've got that bottle in your hands, the question becomes, how do you use it? The options are almost endless. From aromatic diffusers that disperse the oil into the air, to balms and lotions for topical application, the possibilities are vast. But here's where caution and education come into play. Essential oils are potent; they are the concentrated essence of the plant, after all. While a cup of chamomile tea to relax is lovely, a concentrated drop of chamomile essential oil is a different beast altogether. This is why it's important to dilute them properly and perhaps even consult an expert, especially if you're pregnant, nursing, or dealing with any health conditions.

The magic of essential oils also extends to the realm of emotional and spiritual well-being. Some people find that certain oils, like frankincense or myrrh, have a grounding effect, enhancing meditation or spiritual practices. For others, the bright scent of citrus oils like lemon or orange can be uplifting and energizing, great for when you're in need of a little pick-me-up. So, you see, essential oils can be your companions in all walks of life, a kind of olfactory playlist that you can customize based on your mood and needs.

The tale of essential oils is a tapestry woven with threads of history, culture, science, and spirituality. It's a tale that beckons you to become part of it, to experience the rich diversity of plants in a whole new way. As you venture into this aromatic world, remember to do so with both curiosity and caution. After all, essential oils are a gift from the Earth, meant to enrich our lives in countless ways.

But like all gifts of nature, they come with their own set of responsibilities. It's up to us to use them wisely, respectfully, and to remember that in every drop, there's a world of botanical wonder waiting to be discovered.

Of course, let's keep the journey going! While we've been talking about the beauty and appeal of essential oils, it's important to note the scientific research backing their efficacy. Now, while the scientific community has not universally endorsed essential oils as a cure-all, there is a growing body of research that suggests their potential benefits are more than just folklore or hearsay. Studies have looked into the antimicrobial properties of tea tree oil, the anti-inflammatory benefits of lavender, and the stress-reducing effects of bergamot, just to name a few. The blending of ancient wisdom with modern science gives essential oils a sort of dual citizenship in the realms of traditional herbalism and contemporary pharmacology.

But hey, I get it. It's easy to be skeptical when you hear about an oil that claims to do everything from alleviating depression to reducing cellulite. Which brings us to a crucial point: quality matters. Unfortunately, the growing popularity of essential oils has led to a market flooded with synthetic and subpar products. So, how do you sift through the noise? Look for oils that are 100% pure, organic, and sourced responsibly. Labels like "therapeutic grade" are often marketing gimmicks, not standardized certifications. Research the company's reputation, check for transparency in sourcing and testing, and when possible, opt for smaller bottles. Essential oils don't age like fine wine; they can go bad and lose their efficacy.

Now, let's take a detour into the DIY universe, shall we? Because, believe it or not, crafting your own blends can be a rewarding experience. Mixing lavender and chamomile can provide a sleep-enhancing potion, while peppermint and eucalyptus can make for an invigorating blend that may help clear your sinuses. You're like an alchemist in your very own lab, experimenting and discovering the unique combinations that work for you. But as with any scientific endeavor, take notes, be cautious, and maybe wear some gloves.

Speaking of safety, let's get a bit serious here. Essential oils are potent, and their misuse can lead to anything from mild skin irritation to severe toxic reactions. Always dilute the oils appropriately using carrier oils like jojoba, almond, or coconut. A general rule of thumb is to mix 5-6 drops of essential oil per ounce of carrier oil for topical application. And as much as you might love the smell of eucalyptus, keep it away from pets like cats and dogs, for whom many essential oils can be toxic.

Have you ever wondered how essential oils fit into the larger ecosystem? The story is as romantic as it is practical. Essential oils often serve as the plant's defense mechanism against predators, attract pollinators, or even engage in chemical warfare against rival plants. When we extract these oils, we're tapping into the very survival strategies of the plant kingdom. How's that for being connected to nature?

By now, you're armed with a good understanding of the ins and outs of the essential oil world, from its historical roots to its modern-day resurgence, from the intricacies of extraction to the fine print on quality and safety. But remember, the landscape of essential oils is as varied and complex as the plant kingdom itself. You'll find your favorites through trial and error, and perhaps even discover that an oil you'd never considered becomes your go-to for relaxation, focus, or even a spiritual boost. And as you journey through this aromatic and therapeutic world, consider this: you're not just a consumer but a custodian. With each drop, you carry forward a tradition that spans cultures and millennia, blending the wisdom of the ages with the discoveries of today. That, my friend, is a beautiful thing.

We've covered a lot of ground, but there's always more to explore, especially when it comes to the cultural dimensions of essential oils. Have you ever considered the significance of frankincense and myrrh in religious ceremonies? These aromatic resins have been prized for thousands of years, dating back to ancient Egypt and even biblical times. Frankincense was once worth its weight in gold and was among the gifts offered to the baby Jesus, according to Christian tradition. These ancient uses underline the deep cultural and spiritual connections that essential oils can offer.

Speaking of spirituality, essential oils are a significant part of practices like aromatherapy, which aim to heal not just the body, but also the mind and spirit. You'll often find essential oils used in yoga studios, meditation spaces, and other settings where the focus is on holistic well-being. Many people find that specific scents help them reach a deeper level of focus, tranquility, or spiritual connection. If you've ever tried meditating with a diffuser releasing calming lavender or grounding sandalwood, you might know exactly what I'm talking about.

Now, you're probably thinking, "Okay, this all sounds wonderful, but how do I actually use these oils in my daily routine?" Great question! Essential oils can be integrated into your life in various ways, from skincare to house cleaning. For example, a few drops of tea tree oil can enhance your regular facial cleanser, while lemon oil mixed with water makes for a natural and effective surface cleaner. You can even add a couple of drops of your favorite essential oil to a cotton ball and tuck it into your car's air vent for a DIY air freshener.

And, don't forget the culinary possibilities! Some essential oils are food-grade and can add a burst of flavor to dishes. A drop of basil or oregano oil can transform a pasta sauce, and citrus oils like lemon or orange can add zing to desserts. But remember, less is more. These oils are highly concentrated; a single drop can pack a punch.

Now, if you're a parent, you might be wondering about the use of essential oils for children. Pediatricians generally recommend being cautious, as children's skin can be more sensitive to these potent oils. Always consult healthcare professionals and do a patch test before full application. And for the littlest ones, even inhaling certain oils can be too much. So, if you're thinking of using essential oils around kids, consult the experts and proceed with care.

The world of essential oils is an ever-evolving landscape, with ongoing research continually enriching our understanding. Whether you're interested in the chemical components like terpenes and phenols, or the therapeutic potential for conditions like anxiety or insomnia, there's a wealth of information available for you to dive into. Online forums, academic journals, social media groups, and good old-fashioned books can offer various perspectives and insights. Just remember to be discerning and critical when you encounter bold claims or dubious sources.

At this point, you're not just dipping your toes into the essential oil pool—you're doing full-on cannonballs, my friend! And why not? The world of essential oils is as expansive and diverse as the flora from which these oils are extracted. So go ahead, immerse yourself, experiment, and find what resonates with you. Because at the end of the day, your essential oil journey is uniquely your own, and that's the true essence of it all.

Extraction Methods

You see, the plants are like these intricate treasure chests, and inside them are these aromatic compounds just waiting to be unlocked. But getting to the treasure, that's the art and the science of it.

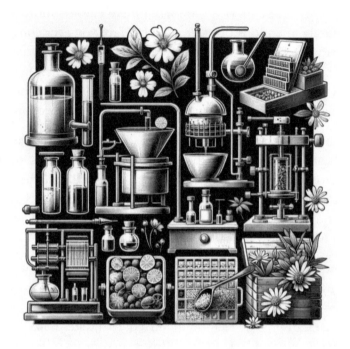

We begin with steam distillation, the most traditional and time-tested method of extraction. Imagine it as a gentle sauna for plants where hot steam passes through plant material, vaporizing the volatile compounds. These vaporized molecules are then channeled into a condensation tube, where they revert back to liquid. The essential oil floats to the top and is separated from the water, much like oil in a vinaigrette. It's a classic method that's been used for centuries, and it's especially great for herbs like lavender and eucalyptus.

Now, if steam distillation is a sauna, then cold pressing is more like a gym workout for the plant. This method is commonly used for citrus fruits like oranges, lemons, and limes. The fruit's rinds are mechanically pressed to squeeze out the oils. Imagine giving an orange a good, hard squeeze and watching those tiny oil droplets spray out—that's essentially what cold pressing achieves but on a much larger scale. If you've ever zested a lemon or smelled your fingers after peeling an orange, you've encountered cold-pressed oils in their most natural form.

For those who are fans of their kitchen gadgets, you'll be thrilled to know that a kind of extraction can happen right in your kitchen with the use of oil maceration. Plant materials like calendula or St. John's Wort can be steeped in a carrier oil over low heat. Picture it as the slow cooking of the essential oil world. The aromatic compounds are gently coaxed into the oil, creating a sumptuous and fragrant infusion. Think of this as the crockpot method of the essential oil world. It's not as concentrated as other methods, but it's a fun and practical way to get into DIY essential oil crafting.

But what about the more exotic and fragile plants, you ask? That's where solvent extraction comes into play. Plants like jasmine and tuberose, which are too delicate for steam distillation, get the royal treatment here. Solvents like hexane or ethanol are used to gently coax out the essential oils without damaging the precious plant materials. It's like a VIP lounge where the most delicate and sensitive of aromatic compounds are treated to an exclusive experience.

Then there's CO2 extraction, the new kid on the block. Think of it as the Tesla of essential oil extraction methods—high-tech and efficient. Carbon dioxide is exposed to high pressure and low temperature, turning it into this unique state that's part liquid, part gas. This 'supercritical' CO2 is then passed through plant material, pulling out even more compounds than steam distillation. The result? A fuller, richer oil that's incredibly pure.

Have you heard of enfleurage? This method is as poetic as its name, used mainly for delicate flowers like jasmine or lily. The petals are laid out on a layer of fat, and over time, the fat absorbs the oil. The process is repeated until the fat is saturated with the oil's fragrance. It's labor-intensive and almost meditative—a true testament to the meticulous care that goes into capturing these elixirs.

And let's not forget about hydrodistillation, particularly effective for waterlogged plants like seaweed or certain types of fungi. The plant material actually sits in water that is then boiled. The steam and oil are captured and condensed just like in steam distillation. This method is like a spa retreat for those plants that love a good soak.

So many methods, each with its own quirks and merits! You might be asking, "Do these methods produce different qualities of oil?" Excellent question. Indeed, they do. Steam-distilled lavender oil, for instance, may have a different chemical profile and therapeutic benefits compared to lavender oil obtained through CO2 extraction. These nuances can make all the difference depending on your needs, whether you're aiming for therapeutic potency or aromatic richness.

As you journey through the aromatic maze of essential oils, understanding these extraction methods can deepen your appreciation for each little bottle's contents. It's like getting to know the backstory of your favorite novel or the behind-the-scenes scoop on a beloved movie. And the more you know, the more empowered you become to make choices that align with your health, ethics, and personal preferences.

So, my aromatic adventurer, are you ready to explore this fragrant world with the curiosity of an alchemist and the wisdom of a sage? The field of extraction is ever-evolving, fusing ancient traditions with modern innovation. Who knows, maybe someday you'll be dabbling in extraction methods we haven't even dreamt of yet!

And there you have it! You're now well-versed in the art and science of essential oil extraction. The plants are calling, and they're ready to share their aromatic secrets. Are you ready to answer?

Now that you've gotten a glimpse into the rich tapestry of extraction methods, let's ponder about the implications. You see, each extraction method isn't just a process; it's a narrative of the plant's journey from earth to bottle. It's a story about preserving the integrity of the plant, capturing its very essence, and bringing its therapeutic goodness into our lives. Just imagine, when you inhale that delightful lavender scent, you're experiencing generations of botanical wisdom and modern scientific innovation, all converging into that one precious moment. It's not just an oil; it's a liquid biography.

But enough waxing poetic, let's talk practicalities. The extraction method not only affects the scent and therapeutic properties of the oil but also its price. For example, rose essential oil can be particularly pricey. Why, you ask? Because it takes an enormous amount of rose petals to produce a single ounce of essential oil. And if it's solvent-extracted to preserve the delicacy of the petals, that involves specialized equipment and expertise, which bumps up the cost. It's a luxury experience akin to sipping a rare vintage wine, each drop a distillation of painstaking labor and pristine growing conditions.

Furthermore, the method of extraction also impacts sustainability. Cold pressing, for instance, is a method that wastes very little of the plant material. It's akin to nose-to-tail eating in the culinary world—nothing is wasted. On the other hand, solvent extraction, while effective for delicate materials, often uses chemicals that can be less eco-friendly. Just as you might opt for locally-sourced, organic produce, choosing essential oils extracted through sustainable methods can be an ethical choice that aligns with your values.

Here's something else to tickle your curiosity. Did you know that certain cultures have their own, unique extraction methods rooted in tradition? For instance, in India, the ancient practice of attar-making involves hydro-distilling flowers into a base of pure sandalwood oil. It's an age-old practice that combines the science of distillation with the art of perfume-making. Imagine this: rows upon rows of copper stills, fired by wood or cow dung, in a quaint, rustic setup that looks like it's been frozen in time. It's a far cry from modern, stainless steel contraptions, and yet it produces attars with a complexity and richness that's unparalleled.

And while we're on the subject of curiosities, let's look back into history. Many ancient civilizations had their own ways of extracting essential oils. The Egyptians, masters of embalming and the cosmetic arts, used methods like maceration and enfleurage long before these processes had fancy names. Their aromatic oils were stored in alabaster jars to keep them potent for years. Even Cleopatra, the ultimate icon of luxury and beauty, was known to have a penchant for rose and neroli oils, undoubtedly obtained through labor-intensive extraction processes. You could say she was the OG (Original Goddess) of essential oil aficionados!

So there you have it, another layer of depth added to your growing knowledge of essential oils. The next time you open a bottle, you won't just smell the oil; you'll sense the landscape from which it came, appreciate the hands that helped bring it to life, and understand the expertise that captured its essence so perfectly. Your relationship with essential oils will be a multi-sensory, multi-dimensional experience, connecting you not just to the plant, but also to a rich lineage of human innovation and Earth's abundant wisdom.

What extraction method has piqued your interest the most? Have you considered how these methods align with your values and needs? The world of essential oils is a lifelong exploration, one where each discovery leads to a deeper question, and each question beckons a more wondrous discovery. Keep exploring, my friend, for the aromatic universe is vast, and you've only just begun to scratch the surface—or should I say, tap the essence?

Understanding how essential oils are extracted gives you a richer appreciation of these fragrant gems. Let's get into the nitty-gritty of different extraction methods, step-by-step.

Steam Distillation
You'll Need: A steam distiller, plant material, water, and collection jars.

1. **Preparation**: Chop your plant material finely to maximize surface area.
2. **Steam Generation**: Fill the bottom chamber of your distiller with water and heat it.
3. **Plant Material**: Place the chopped plant material in the plant chamber.
4. **Steam Through Plant**: Turn on the steam to allow it to pass through the plant chamber.
5. **Condensation**: The steam picks up oil molecules and moves to a condensation chamber.
6. **Separation**: Oil floats on top of water in the condenser; separate the two.

- **Unique Quirks**: This is the most widely used and cost-effective method. However, it's not suitable for heat-sensitive or very delicate plants.
- **Safety Protocols**: Ensure the steam valve is functioning to release pressure. Always use heat-resistant glassware.
- **Ideal Plant Types**: Hardier herbs like rosemary, lavender, and eucalyptus are well-suited for steam distillation.

Cold Pressing (Common for Citrus Oils)
You'll Need: Fresh fruit rinds, a press, and collection jars.
1. **Preparation**: Clean and possibly grate the fruit rinds.
2. **Pressing**: Mechanically press the rinds to squeeze out the oil.
3. **Collect**: Collect the oil and separate it from any juice or water.

Unique Quirks: Primarily used for citrus oils, this method retains the 'freshness' of the fruit. But, it can include some of the fruit's other water-soluble components.
Safety Protocols: Make sure to separate the oil from any juice or water to reduce the risk of microbial growth.
Ideal Plant Types: Citrus fruits like orange, lemon, and lime are the go-to for this method.

Solvent Extraction (Common for Fragile Flowers)
You'll Need: Plant material, a non-polar solvent (like hexane), and evaporation equipment.
1. **Preparation**: Place the delicate plant material on trays.
2. **Solvent Application**: Wash the material with the solvent.
3. **Solution Creation**: The solvent dissolves the plant oils.
4. **Evaporation**: Evaporate the solvent, leaving behind a substance called "concrete."
5. **Alcohol Wash**: Wash the concrete in alcohol to separate waxes and oils.
6. **Final Evaporation**: Evaporate the alcohol to leave just the essential oil.

- **Unique Quirks**: This method is excellent for capturing complex aromas but can result in a less 'pure' oil due to solvent remnants.
- **Safety Protocols**: Only use food-grade or pharmaceutical-grade solvents. Ensure proper ventilation to avoid inhaling fumes.
- **Ideal Plant Types**: Delicate flowers like jasmine, tuberose, and gardenia that can't tolerate heat.

CO2 Extraction
You'll Need: CO_2 extractor, plant material, CO_2 gas, and collection jars.
1. **Preparation**: Load the plant material into the extractor.

2. **CO2**: Inject CO2 gas into the chamber at a high pressure.
3. **Extraction**: The CO2 dissolves the essential oils from the plant.
4. **Decompression**: Release the pressure to separate CO2 and the essential oil.

CO2 Extraction
- **Unique Quirks**: Produces very concentrated oils and is excellent for extracting specific compounds but is more expensive due to the equipment.
- **Safety Protocols**: CO2 extraction should only be done in specialized facilities with the necessary safety measures due to high pressure.
- **Ideal Plant Types**: Plants rich in specialized compounds, such as cloves, young ginger, and black pepper.

Hydrodistillation

You'll Need: Water, plant material, distillation equipment.
1. **Preparation**: Place plant material in a still and cover it with water.
2. **Boiling**: Heat the water until it boils.
3. **Steam Collection**: Collect the steam in a condenser.
4. **Separation**: Separate the essential oil from the water.

- **Unique Quirks**: It's a slower method and can result in slightly 'cooked' or altered aromas due to the direct contact with water.
- **Safety Protocols**: Careful monitoring of temperature and time to avoid destroying the plant material.
- **Ideal Plant Types**: Seeds and roots like coriander seeds and orris root, as well as certain woods and barks.

Enfleurage (Traditional, Less Common)

You'll Need: Fat (animal or vegetable), plant material, glass panes.
1. **Fat Preparation**: Spread a layer of fat on a glass pane.
2. **Plant Material**: Place the plant material on the fat.
3. **Infusion**: Allow the fat to absorb the oils over days or weeks.
4. **Replace**: Replace plant material periodically.
5. **Extraction**: Melt the fat and separate the essential oil.

- **Unique Quirks**: One of the oldest methods and extremely labor-intensive. Great for capturing the full complexity of an aroma, but very expensive.
- **Safety Protocols**: Sanitize all surfaces and containers to prevent bacterial growth in the fat.
- **Ideal Plant Types**: Extremely delicate flowers like lily, tuberose, and certain types of rose that don't respond well to heat or solvents.

Storing and Using Essential Oils Safely

Navigating the world of essential oils is a bit like embarking on a journey through a fragrant forest: each step brings a new scent, a new feeling, and new potential. But like any journey, it's not without its hazards. Sure, you've done the hard work of extraction, but what comes next? The part of the story that often gets overshadowed is storage and safe usage, which, let me tell you, is equally significant.

First of all, imagine spending hours, days, or even weeks crafting the perfect essential oil, only to have it lose its potency or go bad because you stored it in a clear glass bottle under direct sunlight. Devastating, right? Your essential oils are like fine wine; they need the right conditions to flourish. A dark glass bottle is your go-to here. Think of it as the VIP lounge for your oils. The dark glass acts like those swanky, dark sunglasses celebrities wear, protecting the oil from harmful UV rays that could alter its composition.

Speaking of composition, temperature plays a pivotal role as well. A cool, dark place is the equivalent of a five-star hotel for your oils. Don't think your bathroom cabinet counts as 'cool and dark' by the way, because the constant flux of hot showers turns it into a mini-sauna. Not ideal, trust me. A dedicated drawer or cabinet, preferably in a room that stays relatively cool, can be a sanctuary for your oils. If you've got rare or particularly expensive oils, some people even store them in the fridge! Just think about how you'd treat a truffle or a high-quality piece of sashimi; that's the level of care your oils deserve.

Now, we've got storage down, but let's chat about the cap. Or should I say, the caps. Yes, you've got options. The orifice reducer cap is your friend for oils that you'll be dropping into diffusers, mixtures, or just applying a smidge at a time. It limits spillage, and let's face it, there's a kind of satisfaction in getting the perfect drop out, isn't there? Then you have the rollerball cap, ideal for those oils you love to apply directly to your skin—perhaps a lavender or chamomile. Remember, though, not all oils are skin-friendly, so do your homework before you go all in.

It might also be tempting to go "au naturale" and skip any carrier oils when applying directly to the skin. But here's a truth bomb for you: even if you think you've got skin tougher than a rhino, essential oils can be potent. Diluting them in a carrier oil like almond or jojoba not only makes them safer but also allows for more even distribution. Think of the carrier oil as the bread in your avocado toast; sure, the avocado is the star, but you need the bread to hold it all together. A 2-3% dilution is generally safe for adults, which translates to about 2-3 drops of essential oil per teaspoon of carrier oil.

While we're on the topic of safety, let's not forget our furry friends. If you're a pet owner, you might be unaware that some essential oils can be harmful, even toxic, to pets. Cats, for example, can't metabolize citrus oils, and for dogs, high concentrations of tea tree oil can be dangerous. So, before you turn your home into an aromatherapy haven, maybe check whether your choice of essential oils is Fido or Whiskers-friendly.

So you're cautious and you've read up on dilution ratios, and you're pretty confident that you can use your oils safely. Excellent! But, did you ever stop to think about what you're actually inhaling?

There's a reason why certain oils are good for relaxation, while others energize you. That's because these oils have active compounds that interact with your system. It's not just 'smelling nice'; it's chemistry, it's biology—it's almost like a little potion you're concocting.

Which brings me to an often-overlooked point: allergies and medical conditions. I get it, it's exciting to explore the range of oils out there, but it's crucial to remember that these are potent substances. Just because it's natural doesn't mean it's harmless. The same way you wouldn't eat a random plant in the forest, you shouldn't indiscriminately use any oil you get your hands on. Patch tests are your golden ticket to avoid skin irritations or allergic reactions. Dab a little of your diluted oil on a small patch of skin, like the inside of your elbow, and wait 24 hours. No reaction? You're good to go! Any redness or irritation? Well, it's better you found out sooner rather than later.

Now let's circle back to dilution for a moment, especially when it comes to children and babies. Oh boy, this is one area where you have to be extra cautious. Children's skin is more permeable and sensitive than adult skin, and as a result, even a mild essential oil that adults can use undiluted might cause skin irritation in children. Generally, the acceptable dilution ratio for children is 0.5-1%. And for babies? Frankly, unless you're a certified aromatherapist or have consulted with one, it's best to avoid using essential oils altogether for the tiny tots.

To sum up, storing and using essential oils safely is not just about sticking a bottle in a cabinet and calling it a day. It involves understanding the unique needs of each oil, from the bottle it resides in to the way it reacts with your skin and even the air you breathe. Each essential oil comes with its own set of instructions for optimal use and storage. It's a symphony, and you're the conductor. With a little care, a dash of caution, and a sprinkle of knowledge, your essential oil experience will not only be safe but also incredibly rewarding. So, the next time you inhale that soothing waft of lavender or feel the invigorating zing of peppermint, you'll know you've done it right. Keep in mind, the more respectful and knowledgeable you are about these gifts from nature, the more they will give back to you in health and wellness.

Another aspect of using essential oils safely that many people overlook is the practice of "rotating" your oils. Sounds strange? Well, let me elaborate. Overexposure to a single oil or blend can sometimes lead to sensitization, a form of allergic reaction. Rotating your oils is a bit like rotating your crops in farming; it keeps the soil (or in this case, your body) from getting depleted or overexposed to a single element. Consider creating a weekly or bi-weekly rotation to minimize this risk.

And then there's the matter of internal consumption. A few drops of lemon essential oil in your water sounds refreshing, doesn't it? Or perhaps you've heard of adding a drop of peppermint oil to your tea for that extra zing. While it's true that some essential oils can be consumed, this is a slippery slope that we should tread very carefully. You must ensure that the oils you're considering for ingestion are 100% pure, food-grade, and generally recognized as safe (GRAS) by a legitimate body like the FDA. Even then, it's highly recommended to consult a healthcare professional before diving in. It's a bit like taking a new supplement; sure, it's available over the counter, but you wouldn't want to consume it without understanding the potential interactions and side effects.

Okay, so let's consider that you've ticked all the safety boxes. You're storing your oils like a pro, you're applying them like an expert, and you've even got the green light from your healthcare provider for occasional internal use. You might think you've reached the pinnacle of essential oil mastery, right? But wait, there's more. Essential oils, when used in the correct way, can actually complement other healing modalities. For instance, applying lavender oil during a Reiki session can heighten your experience and potential benefits. Similarly, eucalyptus oil can make your sauna session a bit more invigorating. However, it's essential to approach this with knowledge and caution, making sure you're not inadvertently mixing things that shouldn't be mixed. For example, certain oils like grapefruit can interact with medications, making them less effective. Always do your research, and when in doubt, consult a professional.

Now, for those of you thinking of going pro or even semi-pro with your essential oil collection, it's essential to look into good labeling and record-keeping. Think about it: if you're blending your oils or creating your concoctions, it's so easy to forget which bottle contains what. And in the world of essential oils, that's a gamble you don't want to take. Detailed labeling that includes not just the name but also the dilution ratio and the date of blending can save you from potential mishaps. Trust me, "mystery oil" is not a name you want in your collection.

In essence, the journey from oil extraction to safe and effective usage is not as straightforward as it might initially seem. It's an adventure filled with discoveries, a bit of science, and a dash of caution. By being mindful of how you store, apply, and even consume these aromatic wonders, you're not just safeguarding your health, but you're also honoring the essence of the plants from which these oils are derived. This, my friend, is the holistic approach to wellness—conscious, respectful, and infinitely rewarding.

As we wrap this up, I hope you're walking away armed with the knowledge you need to elevate your essential oil experience from novice to pro. But remember, the field is ever-evolving, with new research emerging regularly. Staying updated and continuously learning is part and parcel of the essential oil journey. So go ahead, indulge in the wonders of essential oils, but do it with the wisdom and respect these potent drops of nature truly deserve. Happy oiling!

Let's get practical here. Keeping in mind that essential oils are potent, they require mindful handling and storage. It's kind of like handling your grandma's secret spice mix; a little goes a long way, and it deserves utmost respect and care. So, here are step-by-step instructions on storing and using essential oils safely.

Storing Essential Oils

1. **Choose the Right Container**: Always store your essential oils in glass containers with airtight caps. Avoid using plastic as it can degrade over time. Dark-colored glass like amber or cobalt blue helps to block light, which can deteriorate the oil.
   - **Quirk**: Cobalt blue bottles might make your oils feel like ancient alchemy potions.
   - **Safety Protocol**: Make sure the lid is airtight to prevent any accidental spillage.
   - **Ideal Plant Type**: Good for all types of essential oils.

2. **Temperature Matters**: Store your bottles in a cool, dark place. High temperatures can evaporate and deteriorate the oils.
   - **Quirk**: Some people use wine coolers to maintain the perfect temperature.
   - **Safety Protocol**: Never store near open flames or heat sources.
   - **Ideal Plant Type**: Especially important for citrus oils, which are more susceptible to degradation.
3. **Off the Ground**: Place your essential oil bottles in a wooden storage box or a dedicated shelf, ideally at least 12 inches off the ground.
   - **Quirk**: Some wooden boxes come with little compartments for each oil, which can make you feel like a mixologist.
   - **Safety Protocol**: Make sure the shelf or box is stable and secure.
   - **Ideal Plant Type**: Good for all oils.

Using Essential Oils Safely

1. **Patch Test**: Before applying any oil to larger skin areas, do a patch test to check for allergic reactions. Apply a diluted drop of oil to a small patch of skin on your inner arm and wait 24 hours.
   - **Quirk**: Doing a patch test for each new oil can make you feel like a cautious scientist.
   - **Safety Protocol**: Wash the area immediately if you experience any irritation.
   - **Ideal Plant Type**: Always do this for all essential oils.
2. **Dilute Properly**: Essential oils are highly concentrated and should be diluted using a carrier oil like jojoba or coconut oil before topical application.
   - **Quirk**: You can become a blending artist, trying different combinations of oils and carriers for various effects.
   - **Safety Protocol**: The general guideline is 2-3 drops of essential oil per tablespoon of carrier oil.
   - **Ideal Plant Type**: Especially critical for "hot" oils like cinnamon and clove.
3. **Inhalation Methods**: If using an essential oil diffuser, follow the manufacturer's instructions.
   - **Quirk**: Some diffusers come with lights and sounds, providing a complete sensory experience.
   - **Safety Protocol**: Limit diffusion to 30-60 minutes at a time to avoid overwhelming the senses.
   - **Ideal Plant Type**: Oils like lavender and chamomile are great for relaxation.
4. **Oral Consumption**: If you're considering taking essential oils internally, consult a healthcare professional first.
   - **Quirk**: A drop of peppermint oil can replace a breath mint but consult a professional first.
   - **Safety Protocol**: Use food-grade oils and follow professional guidelines for dosage.
   - **Ideal Plant Type**: Generally, only common culinary oils like peppermint and lemon are considered for internal use, and even then, it's a subject of debate.

By following these practical steps and safety protocols, you'll not only ensure that your oils stay potent for longer but also that you're using them in a way that maximizes their benefits while minimizing risks. So, here's to your aromatic and therapeutic journey with essential oils!

Chapter 5: The Art of Making Tinctures

Alright, let's dive right into the enchanted world of tinctures, shall we? You know, tinctures are like the unsung heroes of the herbal medicine cabinet. They're versatile, potent, and—believe it or not—super easy to make. Imagine capturing the essence of an herb, holding its therapeutic powers captive in a little glass dropper bottle, ready to come to your rescue whenever you need it. That's a tincture for you. Essentially, a tincture is a concentrated herbal extract. The word may sound fancy, but don't let it intimidate you. Tinctures are as commonplace in herbal medicine as smoothies are in health food stores!

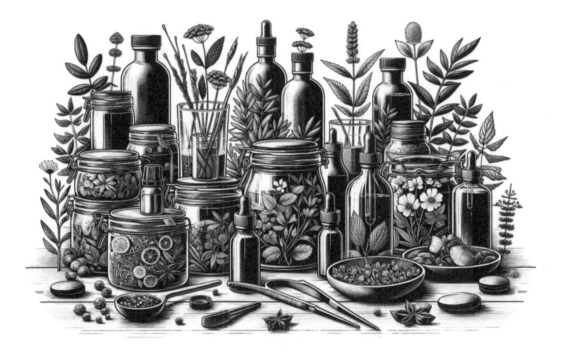

Okay, now how do you go about capturing the very spirit of a plant? Picture this: you're soaking a handful of your chosen herb in a jar of alcohol, shaking it occasionally and giving it some sweet talk. Yes, really, some folks believe in communicating with the plants they're working with; call it plant whispering if you like! You let this soak or macerate for a good couple of weeks, and voila! You've got yourself a liquid herbal ally, my friend.

The process might sound rudimentary, but here's where the magic happens. The alcohol acts as a solvent, pulling out the essential components of the herb. We're talking alkaloids, flavonoids, and all those other scientific-sounding words that basically mean "the good stuff." And you don't have to limit yourself to alcohol; vinegar or vegetable glycerin work too, especially if you're teetotal or need to administer it to children.

Now comes the part that makes you feel like a true apothecarist—straining and bottling your creation. Using a cheesecloth or fine mesh strainer, you'll separate the liquid from the plant matter. This liquid gold, my friend, is your tincture. Bottle it up in amber dropper bottles, label them meticulously, and you're all set.

So how do you use this bottled magic? The beauty of tinctures lies in their versatility. Depending on what herbs you use, tinctures can serve a multitude of purposes. Got trouble sleeping? A few drops of valerian root tincture might just send you off to dreamland. Need a quick immunity boost? Echinacea tincture to the rescue! And when it comes to dosages, remember, these are potent potions; usually, a dropperful or two is all you need.

But before you go full-on potion master, a word of caution. Tinctures are powerful stuff, and while they are derived from plants, they can still interact with medications or conditions you may have. It's always wise to consult with a healthcare professional about proper dosages and any potential interactions. Consider this step as you gathering your allies before embarking on any epic quest.

Alright, there you have it—a whirlwind tour of what tinctures are, how to make them, and how to use them safely. Imagine, all this potent plant power can be yours to command, right from your kitchen! Are you feeling the herbalist vibes yet? Because I think you're more than ready to dive into this tincture-making journey. Happy tincturing!

What are Tinctures?

The name itself sounds like something out of an alchemist's handbook, doesn't it? Well, in a way, it's not far from the truth. If you've ever been intrigued by the idea of capturing the very essence of a plant, its soul if you will, then welcome to the world of tinctures. These are highly concentrated liquid extracts that manage to bottle up the medicinal properties of herbs and plants. Imagine having the power of an entire garden in a small amber bottle on your kitchen shelf—that's what tinctures offer you.

You see, herbs have been our companions through millennia. Every culture has its treasure trove of herbal remedies, those age-old secrets passed down through generations. What tinctures do is concentrate that ancient wisdom into a form that's not just potent but also convenient. Imagine you're coming down with a cold. Wouldn't it be nice to reach for a dropper of echinacea tincture instead of boiling pots of tea or grinding herbs for a remedy? A few drops and you've got yourself a powerful ally in fighting off that pesky virus.

And don't think for a moment that tinctures are some kind of newfangled invention. Oh no, these have a long history dating back hundreds of years. Medieval apothecaries were known for their extensive use of tinctures. These were the pharmacists of their time, blending, extracting, and distilling plants in various forms, including tinctures. They used alcohol, vinegar, or other solvents to extract the medicinal compounds from herbs. Over time, this practice has been refined but the basic principle remains the same: isolating and preserving the most beneficial elements of plants.

So how are these liquid miracles made? The process is almost poetic in its simplicity. You take your chosen herb—let's say lavender for its calming effects—and you steep it in a solvent like alcohol. Picture the alcohol as this enthusiastic interviewer coaxing out the deepest secrets from a wise elder—that elder being the lavender. The alcohol draws out the essential oils, flavonoids, alkaloids, and other beneficial compounds from the plant matter. These compounds are what give the plant its medicinal or therapeutic properties. Over a period of weeks, the plant matter imbues the alcohol with its essence, and what you're left with is a highly concentrated liquid.

It's like having the cliff notes of the plant—short, powerful, and to the point. Just a few drops under your tongue, added to a glass of water, or even incorporated into your cooking, and you've harnessed the herb's potential benefits. And because they're so concentrated, tinctures often act faster than other herbal preparations. It's almost as if the plant's healing energy is delivered in a more direct, unadulterated form.

There's a tincture for almost everything under the sun—from digestive issues and sleep problems to stress relief and immune support. Whether it's the soothing touch of chamomile, the invigorating burst of ginseng, or the antimicrobial might of garlic, there's a tincture out there tailored to your needs.

But wait, let's not get carried away. While tinctures are relatively safe, they are still potent extractions. You need to be cautious with dosages and, of course, it's always good to have a chat with a healthcare professional, especially if you're pregnant, nursing, or on certain medications.

So there you have it—the essence of what tinctures are, captured much like how a tincture captures the essence of a plant. It's a beautiful synergy, don't you think? From gardens and apothecary shelves of yore to your modern-day kitchen, tinctures bridge the old and the new, giving you the means to take control of your well-being, one drop at a time. Now, doesn't that make you want to start your own little tincture collection?

So we've established that tinctures are these powerful elixirs that carry within them the very soul of a plant, but have you ever wondered how exactly they fit into the grand tapestry of herbal medicine? You see, tinctures are just one piece of the puzzle. The world of herbal remedies is vast and varied, ranging from teas and poultices to oils and capsules. But when it comes to sheer convenience and potency, tinctures are hard to beat.

Think about how fast-paced our lives have become. We're always on the go, hustling from one task to another. In this whirlwind lifestyle, who has the time to brew herbal teas or prepare elaborate remedies? Enter tinctures. They're like the fast food of herbal medicine—quick, easy, and effective—except they're actually good for you! A few drops can be taken straight or easily mixed into a drink, offering you a no-fuss way to incorporate herbal goodness into your day.

Another fascinating aspect of tinctures is their longevity. Because they're alcohol-based, they have a long shelf-life. In some cases, tinctures can last for years if stored correctly. This is a stark contrast to fresh herbs, which spoil relatively quickly. So, in essence, a tincture is like a time capsule. It captures the potency of the herb at its peak and preserves it for your use, long after the plant itself would have withered and lost its potency.

Now, let's talk about the diversity of tinctures, shall we? There's literally a world of plants out there to choose from, each with its own unique profile of medicinal compounds. Ever heard of milk thistle? It's a great detoxifier for your liver. Or what about passionflower, which has been shown to help with anxiety and sleep disorders? Then there's the good old ginger tincture that aids in digestion and can help alleviate nausea. The possibilities are endless, limited only by the types of plants you can access and your willingness to experiment.

When it comes to customization, tinctures are the epitome of personalization in herbal medicine. You can mix different tinctures together to create your own bespoke remedies tailored to your specific needs. Picture this: you're feeling a bit under the weather, a sore throat is bothering you, and you're feeling more anxious than usual about a looming deadline. Instead of taking separate remedies for each issue, you could create a blend from echinacea, lemon balm, and lavender tinctures. Voila! You've crafted your own personalized wellness cocktail.

And it's not just the physical ailments that tinctures can address. Many herbs have mood-boosting or calming properties. St. John's Wort is popularly used for mild depression, and Valerian root is like nature's Valium, providing relief from anxiety and helping you sleep. So you see, tinctures can offer holistic care, nurturing not just your body but also your mind.

In a world where quick-fix pharmaceuticals are often sought after, tinctures serve as a poignant reminder of the enduring power of nature. They remind us that before there were labs, there were gardens. Before there were pharmacists, there were herbalists. And before there were synthetic drugs, there were plants—humble, yet filled with the incredible power to heal and nurture.

Tinctures are a celebration of that primal, sacred relationship between humans and the plant kingdom. They encapsulate millennia of human wisdom, tradition, and most importantly, a deep reverence for the healing power of nature. So the next time you hold a small bottle of tincture, know that you're not just holding a remedy, but a rich, liquid tapestry of history, culture, and the untamed wonders of the natural world.

I hope this extended dive into the world of tinctures adds another layer of understanding and fascination for you. So, are you ready to bring this ancient form of herbal magic into your modern life?

Tincturing Process

Let's embark on a fascinating journey to explore the intricate art of making tinctures. Picture yourself as a modern-day alchemist, part scientist and part artist, concocting magic in liquid form. There's something deeply rewarding about creating your own herbal tinctures; it's as if you're taking an active role in your wellness story, and guess what? It's not as complicated as it might seem. With the right ingredients and a dash of patience, you're well on your way to crafting your own herbal remedies.

So, where do we begin? Yes, ingredients. The first step is to choose the plant or plants you want to tincture. For novices, it's a good idea to start with something familiar and abundantly available. Think of herbs like chamomile, which is great for relaxation, or peppermint, wonderful for digestion. But don't just grab any plant and dunk it in alcohol. Identifying the right plant species is crucial for both efficacy and safety. A simple mistake in identification can, at best, make your tincture useless and, at worst, be harmful.

Once you've selected your herb, the next crucial decision involves the type of solvent you'll use. In layman's terms, a solvent is what extracts the medicinal compounds from the plant, and in the case of most tinctures, that solvent is alcohol. However, the percentage of alcohol can vary depending on the plant. Some herbs require a higher alcohol content to effectively extract their medicinal components, while others do just fine with a lower percentage. This is where a little bit of research can go a long way. A general rule of thumb is that harder, woodier parts like roots and bark require a higher percentage of alcohol, while softer parts like leaves and flowers can do with less.

Now let's talk about the 'maceration' process, the heart of tincture-making. Don't let the technical term intimidate you; maceration is essentially just soaking the plant material in the solvent to extract its goodness. It's like making tea but in slow motion and with alcohol. You take your chosen plant parts, chop them finely to increase the surface area for better extraction, and then submerge them in alcohol. This mixture is usually kept in a sealed jar and needs to be stored in a cool, dark place for an extended period—usually around four to six weeks. Every day or so, give the jar a good shake to help the extraction process along.

You might be wondering why it takes so long. Well, patience is a virtue, especially in herbal medicine. The extended soaking time ensures that a broad spectrum of the plant's medicinal compounds are extracted. And don't worry about the alcohol content; while it's true that you're consuming a few drops of alcohol when you take a tincture, the amount is so minuscule that it's generally not a concern for most people. However, if you're avoiding alcohol for any reason, alternatives like vegetable glycerin can be used, though they might not be as effective in extracting all the beneficial compounds from the herb.

When the maceration period is over, it's time for the grand unveiling. Strain the plant material from the liquid, and what remains is your tincture. This should be stored in a dark glass bottle to protect it from light, which can degrade its potency. Some people even like to use dropper bottles for easy administration.

But wait, there's more. You see, tincturing isn't a one-size-fits-all process. Different herbs have different quirks, and as you gain more experience, you'll find that you can tweak the basic tincturing process to better suit specific plants. For instance, some herbs are better tinctured fresh, while others should be dried first. Then there are some that benefit from a double maceration process for an even stronger tincture. Yes, it's a labor of love, but one that pays off generously in terms of both wellness and the satisfaction of having created something invaluable.

If you thought the world of tinctures is a mere subcategory in the broad spectrum of herbal medicine, you'd be mistaken. It's a universe unto itself, one filled with endless possibilities for exploration and experimentation. The combinations of plants, the tweaking of alcohol percentages, the fine-tuning of maceration times—all these offer an endless canvas upon which you can paint your own unique blend of wellness.

In summary, the process of tincturing is like a dance—a harmonious interplay between the plant and the solvent, one coaxing out the best qualities of the other. Each step, from choosing the right plant and solvent to the maceration period, is a verse in a poetic ode to nature's healing power. The end result? A potent, personalized remedy that's imbued not just with the essence of the plant, but also with your intent, care, and reverence for the natural world. And that, my friend, is nothing short of magical.

So, are you ready to roll up your sleeves and dive into the intoxicating world of tinctures? Trust me, once you start, it's a lifelong journey of discovery, one where each tincture you create is a stepping stone to a deeper understanding of both plants and yourself.

Let's discuss the concept of 'ratios' in tincturing. When making a tincture, you can't just haphazardly toss herbs into a jar and cover them with alcohol; well, technically you could, but that wouldn't be very effective. Understanding the ratio of herb to solvent is crucial for achieving a potent tincture. Usually, this ratio is expressed in terms like 1:5 or 1:2, where the first number refers to the volume of the herb, and the second number refers to the volume of the solvent. For instance, a 1:5 ratio would mean that for every one part of herb, you'll need five parts of the solvent. Measuring can be done by weight or volume, though many herbalists prefer weight for greater accuracy. But don't stress too much; while precision is good, herbalism is also forgiving of some approximations.

Moreover, these ratios can be adjusted depending on what you're tincturing. A super potent herb may require less solvent, while something milder may need a higher volume of alcohol to capture its essence effectively. The ratios also vary depending on whether you're using fresh or dried herbs, as dried herbs are more concentrated.

Now, let's delve into 'folk method' vs 'standardized method.' The folk method is more intuitive. You simply fill a jar about two-thirds full with your herb, then pour the alcohol over it until the jar is full. Many home herbalists prefer this method because it's straightforward and requires no calculations. On the other hand, the standardized method involves using precise measurements and sometimes even scales to ensure a specific ratio of herb to alcohol. This method is particularly useful for those who are making tinctures for medicinal purposes where exact dosages are crucial.

As you grow more experienced in your tincturing adventures, you might even delve into 'multi-herb tinctures,' which are exactly what they sound like: tinctures made from more than one type of herb. Crafting these requires a good understanding of each herb's properties and how they'll interact not just with the solvent but also with each other. It's like being a chef, crafting a gourmet meal; each ingredient needs to complement the others, enhancing the overall effectiveness of the tincture.

Another layer of sophistication can be added by considering the 'moon cycles' while making your tinctures. Some herbalists swear by starting their tincture on a new moon and straining it on a full moon. While there's limited scientific evidence supporting this practice, many find a deeper spiritual connection to their work by aligning it with the lunar phases.

There's a joy in mastering the details, in finding the nuances that let you make each tincture uniquely your own. After all, the beauty of tincturing lies in its melding of science and art, measurement and intuition, potency and grace. Each jar you fill becomes both a sanctuary of healing and a testament to your growing skill and wisdom.

So there you have it, the tincturing process in all its glory, teeming with opportunities for both the novice and the seasoned herbalist to explore and grow. With each tincture you make, you're not just extracting plant compounds; you're also distilling a richer understanding of this ancient practice, and perhaps, gaining a deeper insight into your own healing journey.

Feel inspired? I hope so. The world of tinctures is vast and vibrant, waiting for you to dive in and discover its many wonders.

Let's distill the tincturing process into a practical, step-by-step guide. While I'm at it, I'll sprinkle in some unique quirks, safety protocols, and tips on selecting the ideal plants for different methods.

The Folk Method

Step-by-Step:
1. **Select Your Herb**: Choose fresh or dried herbs. Fresh is generally better for plants high in water content.
2. **Prepare the Jar**: Use a sterilized, dry glass jar.
3. **Herb Placement**: Fill the jar about two-thirds full with your herb of choice.
4. **Add Solvent**: Pour high-proof alcohol (80-100 proof for fresh herbs, 90-100 for dried) over the herbs until the jar is full.
5. **Seal and Shake**: Tighten the lid and give the jar a good shake.
6. **Store**: Keep it in a cool, dark place for 4-6 weeks.
7. **Shake Daily**: Remember to shake it every day.
8. **Strain**: After 4-6 weeks, strain out the herbs, and your tincture is ready!

Unique Quirks:
• Folk method enthusiasts often start their tincture on a new moon and strain it on a full moon.

Safety Protocols:
• Always use food-grade alcohol.
• If you're pregnant, nursing, or have a medical condition, consult a healthcare provider.

Ideal Plant Types:
• Mint, chamomile, and lavender are excellent choices for beginners.

The Standardized Method

Step-by-Step:
1. **Weigh Your Herb**: Use a scale to weigh the herb precisely.
2. **Measure Solvent**: Based on your herb-to-alcohol ratio, measure the amount of solvent needed.
3. **Combine**: Add the herb and solvent to a sterilized glass jar.
4. **Seal and Store**: Seal the jar tightly and store it in a dark, cool place.
5. **Shake Daily**: Shake the jar daily for 4-6 weeks.
6. **Strain and Store**: After the steeping time, strain out the herbs.

Unique Quirks:
- Some people use amber glass bottles with droppers for more precise dosing.

Safety Protocols:
- Be extra careful about the herb-to-alcohol ratio, especially for potent herbs.

Ideal Plant Types:
- Roots and barks, like ginseng and willow, are often tinctured using this method for precise dosing.

The Glycerin Method (Non-Alcoholic)

Step-by-Step:
1. **Select Herb and Solvent**: Choose your herb and glycerin as the solvent.
2. **Combine**: Add herb and glycerin to a glass jar, using a 1:3 ratio.
3. **Seal and Store**: Close the jar and store it in a dark place for 4-6 weeks.
4. **Shake Daily**: Yes, again with the shaking. It's crucial.
5. **Strain**: Strain out the herb material, and voila!

Unique Quirks:
- Glycerin tinctures have a sweet taste, making them kid-friendly.

Safety Protocols:
- Use food-grade, vegetable glycerin.

Ideal Plant Types:
- Lemon balm and ginger are popular choices due to the sweet solvent.

The Vinegar Method (Non-Alcoholic)

Step-by-Step:
1. **Select Herb and Solvent**: Choose your herb and use apple cider vinegar as the solvent.
2. **Combine**: Like the glycerin method, a 1:3 ratio works well.
3. **Seal, Store, and Shake**: Store it in a dark place and remember to shake daily for 4-6 weeks.
4. **Strain**: Strain the herbs out, and your vinegar tincture is ready.

Unique Quirks:
- Vinegar tinctures have a tangy flavor and are often used in cooking.

Safety Protocols:
- Opt for organic, unpasteurized apple cider vinegar.

Ideal Plant Types:
- Herbs like rosemary and thyme are ideal for vinegar tinctures.

There you have it! A detailed, step-by-step guide to different methods of making tinctures, complete with unique quirks, safety tips, and ideal plant suggestions. Happy tincturing!

Uses and Dosages

Of course, diving into the world of tinctures would be incomplete without understanding their uses and dosages, right? Imagine you've just crafted a beautiful tincture, maybe from calming lavender or invigorating ginger, and it's sitting on your kitchen shelf like a trophy. But this is no trophy to be stared at; it's a functional tool for well-being that's itching to be used.

Let's start by debunking the notion that tinctures are some mystical, ambiguous liquid only meant for the most hardcore herbalists. In reality, they are quite user-friendly and versatile, making them a fantastic starting point for anyone wanting to weave herbal medicine into their daily life. Tinctures are highly concentrated, meaning that a small dose goes a long way. You're not going to have to chug half a bottle to see an effect; we're talking drops, not gulps.

For example, a tincture made from a powerhouse herb like Echinacea can be a game-changer during flu season. Just a few drops under the tongue at the first sign of a scratchy throat can kickstart your immune response. Or, perhaps you've brewed a peppermint tincture, a soothing digestive aid, perfect after an indulgent meal. A small dose can ease the feeling of fullness and even tackle symptoms of irritable bowel syndrome. But, as wonderful as tinctures are, it's crucial to understand that more doesn't always mean better. A concentrated extract of any herb still carries all its complexities, including the potential for adverse reactions or interactions with other medications.

Dosage is a crucial aspect, often individualized based on factors like age, health conditions, and the strength of the tincture. While general guidelines can be useful, it's advisable to consult a healthcare provider, particularly for those who are pregnant, nursing, or under any medication. Tinctures can be surprisingly potent, and what works for your neighbor Joe may not be suitable for you. Typically, the dosage information is either available on the packaging or through the resource you've used to create the tincture, especially if it's a trusted herbal book or an experienced herbalist's recipe.

The concept of "start low and go slow" is like the golden rule of tincture dosages. For adults, starting with a small dose like 1-2 ml once or twice a day is a commonly recommended amount. Observe how your body reacts, and then gradually adjust the dosage. Some people find it useful to maintain a journal, noting down any changes in symptoms or overall well-being.

It's also worth mentioning that tinctures are not just for swallowing. They can be used topically for issues like skin infections or even as a scalp treatment for dandruff. And for culinary enthusiasts, some tinctures like vanilla or mint are excellent additions to recipes, adding both flavor and health benefits to your dishes.

It's fascinating to see how the tincture dosages and applications differ from one herb to another. While adaptogenic herbs like ashwagandha are generally taken over extended periods to help the body adapt to stress, fast-acting herbs like valerian are better suited for acute situations, like insomnia. Likewise, herbs that have a cumulative effect, such as turmeric, are best when consistently integrated into your routine over time.

Now, let's talk about some age-old practices that come with their own sets of traditions and wisdom. In Traditional Chinese Medicine and Ayurveda, the dosage and application of herbal tinctures might vary significantly, often incorporating elements like the patient's constitution, current imbalances, and even the season. These systems may use specific synergistic blends of herbs, designed to balance out the stronger effects of one herb with the milder effects of another. In these contexts, the role of a skilled practitioner is invaluable for determining the appropriate dosages and combinations.

For children and pets, the dosages need to be adjusted accordingly, often scaled down considerably. In the case of children, herbalists generally recommend calculating the dosage based on the child's weight, employing what's known as Clark's Rule. The formula is: (child's weight in pounds / 150) x adult dosage = child's dosage. As always, when it comes to kids and pets, it's crucial to consult a healthcare provider or a vet for specific guidance.

It's not just about what you take; it's also about how you take it. Some tinctures, especially those made from bitter herbs, are more effective when taken on an empty stomach. This can stimulate the production of digestive enzymes and gastric juices. However, some people find that certain tinctures, like those made from spicy or warming herbs, can be a bit hard on the stomach and are better taken with food.

Here's where we touch on a point that's often glossed over: the importance of mindful consumption. In our hurry to get results, it's easy to overlook the deeper relationship we're forming with these plants. Each time you use a tincture, take a moment to smell it, savor its flavor, and appreciate the natural bounty it came from. This mindfulness not only enhances your experience but can also sharpen your awareness of how your body responds to different herbs, making you more attuned to finding the perfect dose for yourself.

So there you have it—a sprawling landscape of the uses and dosages of herbal tinctures, from the nitty-gritty of dosing to the nuances of different herbal traditions. It's a journey, really, one that can make you an active participant in your own well-being, empowering you to take control of your health naturally. Remember, the world of herbal tinctures is as vast as it is ancient, offering a wealth of opportunities to improve your quality of life. All it takes is a dropper and a dash of curiosity.

While we've touched on some key points about dosage and applications, there are further intricacies worth exploring. The versatility of tinctures also means you can use them in a range of situations. For example, you might turn to a chamomile tincture to calm down before a big presentation at work, or perhaps rely on a ginger tincture to ease motion sickness during a long car ride. And it's not just about physical symptoms—many people find that tinctures made from herbs like St. John's Wort or lemon balm can have a significantly positive impact on mood and mental well-being.

In line with the age-old adage that "prevention is better than cure," some herbalists even recommend 'tonic tinctures,' designed for daily consumption to maintain overall health and prevent illness. These usually contain herbs that are considered adaptogens, which help the body adapt to stress and maintain equilibrium. Think of herbs like ginseng, holy basil, or rhodiola. However, it's good to keep in mind that even tonic tinctures shouldn't be consumed endlessly. Giving yourself a break allows your body to process the herbs and can also help prevent developing a tolerance to the tincture's effects.

Let's talk about the delivery method a bit more. You know how some people cringe at the idea of swallowing pills? Well, tinctures are a brilliant alternative, offering a less intrusive and often more immediate effect. You can place a few drops directly under the tongue, known as sublingual administration, for rapid absorption into the bloodstream. This is especially beneficial for herbs intended to have quick effects, such as rescue remedy or feverfew for migraines. The alcohol base in tinctures ensures that the active compounds in the herb are easily and quickly absorbed, making it an efficient mode of delivery.

Now, while the sublingual method is quick and effective, not everyone enjoys the strong taste of concentrated herbs. In that case, you can always add your tincture to a little water or juice to make it more palatable. Some people get creative and include tinctures in their smoothies, teas, or even soups! But keep in mind that mixing the tincture with food or drink may slightly delay its effects.

Speaking of taste, let's not overlook the role of flavor in herbal medicine. The taste itself can offer clues about the tincture's effects. For instance, bitter herbs like dandelion or wormwood can stimulate digestion, while sweet herbs like licorice often act as adaptogens. Many traditional medicine systems, including Ayurveda and Traditional Chinese Medicine, use the 'doctrine of signatures,' an age-old belief that the taste, shape, and color of an herb give indications of its therapeutic properties. While modern science doesn't fully subscribe to this idea, there is a sense of intuitive wisdom to it that many find valuable.

A common question often posed is about the alcohol content in tinctures. Yes, most tinctures are alcohol-based because alcohol is a powerful solvent that efficiently extracts the active compounds from herbs. But if you're avoiding alcohol for any reason, there are alternatives like glycerin-based or vinegar-based tinctures. However, it's essential to note that these may not be as potent or have a shorter shelf-life compared to their alcohol-based counterparts.

Also, for those who are managing chronic conditions like diabetes, hypertension, or any hormonal imbalances, remember that while tinctures can be an excellent supplementary treatment, they should not replace any medication or treatment plan you're currently on, unless advised by a qualified healthcare provider. Always keep your medical team in the loop about any herbal remedies you're considering.

In closing, it's worth noting that the realm of tinctures is a fascinating intersection of art, science, tradition, and personal experience. With the multitude of herbs available, each with its unique profile of active compounds, the possibilities are nearly endless. There's a sense of empowerment that comes from understanding not just the 'how,' but also the 'why' behind tincture dosages and uses. You become not just a consumer, but an informed participant in your wellness journey. The first time you experience the tangible benefits of a tincture you've carefully selected or even made yourself, it's nothing short of magical—a real-life potion that brings the incredible world of plants right into the palm of your hand.

Chapter 6: Brewing Herbal Infusions

Picture this: a cozy morning where you're sipping a fragrant cup of herbal tea, your body filling up with warmth and your mind feeling as clear as the morning sky. Or imagine that it's late at night, and a mug of a relaxing infusion prepares you for a restful sleep. But these infusions and decoctions are not just about aromatic experiences or soul-soothing rituals; they also pack a punch when it comes to health benefits.

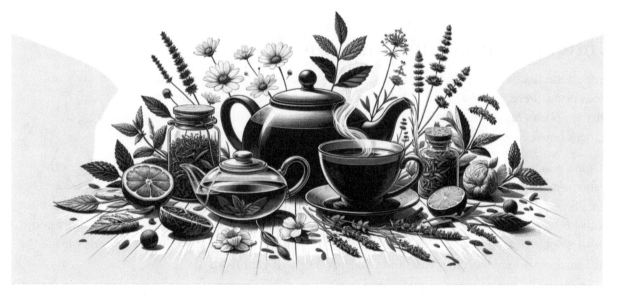

If you've been thinking that infusions and decoctions are just fancy words for herbal teas, well, you're not entirely wrong. However, there are distinctions, and these distinctions are rooted in the methods used to extract the beneficial compounds from our chosen herbs. Infusions are generally lighter and are great for leaves and flowers, whereas decoctions are typically used for tougher, woody materials like bark and roots. It's the alchemy of water and herbs—each method allows the water to become a medium that captures the essence, both flavor-wise and medicinally, of the plant materials.

And it's not a one-size-fits-all thing. The potency of your concoction will depend on the ratio of water to herbs, the temperature, and the steeping time, among other factors. A higher ratio of herbs doesn't always mean a better infusion; sometimes, it can even be overpowering. Finding the perfect balance is like creating a personalized potion, one that's attuned to your body's needs. And don't worry, we'll go through some common techniques and ratios to get you started on the right foot.

Now, what's truly amazing is that there's an almost endless variety of herbs you can use. From popular choices like chamomile and peppermint to exotic names like ashwagandha and skullcap, each herb brings its own unique health benefits and flavors to the table. So, in the mood for some mental clarity? A rosemary or ginkgo infusion might be your best friend. Dealing with digestive issues? A simple ginger or peppermint tea could do wonders.

But here's where it gets even more exciting. You can mix and match! Yes, you can combine herbs to suit your taste and health requirements. A blend of lavender and chamomile can create a super-soothing tonic, while a mix of echinacea and elderberry could be your go-to concoction during cold and flu season.

So grab your favorite cup, and let's delve into this journey through the versatile and enriching universe of herbal infusions and decoctions. Whether you're a beginner looking to explore or a seasoned herbal enthusiast aiming to refine your craft, this chapter will provide you with the insights, techniques, and inspiration you need to enrich your life through the transformative power of plants. Cheers to that!

Understanding Infusions and Decoctions

They sound like terms straight out of a wizard's spellbook, don't they? But trust me, there's no hocus pocus here, just good old botanical magic, steeped in tradition, science, and a touch of artistry. So let's take a close look at what they are, how they're different, and why knowing the nuances between the two can make a significant difference in your herbal journey.

Imagine you're an alchemist in your own cozy kitchen. You're surrounded by jars of dried herbs, fresh sprigs from your garden, and various other botanicals. You're ready to extract their essences into a liquid form so you can ingest them easily and absorb their benefits. Here, your role is not just about brewing a cuppa; you're engaging in a medicinal practice that spans thousands of years and countless cultures. How you choose to brew—either by infusion or decoction—depends on the plant material you're working with, and what you hope to gain from it.

Let's start with infusions. When we talk about infusions, we're generally referring to the act of steeping lighter plant materials like leaves, flowers, or seeds in hot water. Think of chamomile flowers, peppermint leaves, or fennel seeds. It's like making tea, but with a more deliberate intention of pulling out beneficial compounds. The water should be hot, but not boiling, as boiling water can destroy some of the more delicate compounds. These steeped mixtures are best consumed fresh to get the most benefits, but they can also be refrigerated for a day or two. You're usually looking at a ratio of about a handful of herbs to a cup of water, but this is where your personal touch can come in. You could add a little more of this or a tad less of that, depending on your health needs and flavor preferences. You might also consider covering the infusion while it steeps to keep the volatile oils from escaping—those oils are often where the plant stores its most potent medicinal properties.

Now, on to decoctions. These are the heavy-duty siblings of infusions. While infusions are like a leisurely walk in the park, decoctions are like a rigorous hike up a mountain. Decoctions are designed to extract the deeper, harder-to-reach compounds found in more rigid and woody plant materials like roots, bark, and stems. You'll need to simmer these materials in water over low heat for a longer period, usually about 20-45 minutes. You can't rush this process; it's a slow release of potent compounds that wouldn't be as accessible through a simple infusion. The plant-to-water ratio for decoctions is typically more generous, as you'll want to extract as much goodness as possible. These preparations are more concentrated, and they can be stored for a bit longer, though fresh is still best.

Both infusions and decoctions can be consumed on their own, added to foods, or even used topically depending on the herb and your needs. However, while infusions are generally safe to consume freely, you might need to be more careful with decoctions. Because of their concentration, they can be potent and should be consumed in moderation.

Now, why is it essential to distinguish between these two methods? It boils down to maximizing the medicinal value of the plant materials. Some compounds are delicate and will break down if subjected to prolonged heat, making them ideal candidates for infusions. On the flip side, the resilient compounds that reside in roots and barks need the alchemy of slow-cooked decoctions to be fully released. The nature of the plant dictates the method, and knowing the difference allows you to extract the maximum benefits from your herbal preparations.

That's not to say you can't get creative! Once you've mastered the basics, you can experiment. Some herbalists like to make a decoction first, then add lighter plant materials for an infusion, effectively making a combined brew. It's an infusion-decoction hybrid, if you will. It's like layering flavors in a complex dish; each process brings out a different set of compounds and contributes to the final, multi-faceted result.

Let me share a little secret—there are no hard and fast rules in this herbal alchemy. The guidelines are there to help you get started, but your intuition, built from experience and experimentation, will be your best guide. As you become more familiar with various herbs, their properties, and how they interact with your body, you'll find yourself naturally gravitating towards specific plants, combinations, and methods. This is where the artistry comes in.

So go ahead, channel your inner alchemist, and get brewing. Whether you're gently steeping a fragrant mix of lavender and chamomile or simmering a potent decoction of ginger and turmeric roots, you're participating in an age-old tradition of harnessing the power of plants for well-being. Each brew is a celebration, a remedy, and a nourishing elixir, customized by the most qualified person—you.

Now that we've dipped our toes into the waters of infusions and decoctions, let's wade a little deeper into some of the fascinating details that make these methods unique. There's a lot to unpack, from the energy you bring into the brewing process to the various textures, colors, and flavors that each herb imparts. It's not just about the active compounds but also about the symphony they create when combined, not just within the brew but also within you.

For example, ever noticed how the simple act of holding a warm mug of herbal tea can elevate your mood? Or how the aroma wafting from a simmering decoction can fill your space with a sense of grounding or invigorate your senses? That's the holistic magic of these practices, my friend. The herbs aren't just working on a biochemical level, but they're also interacting with your senses, emotions, and even your spiritual self.

Let's say you're making a cup of chamomile infusion. You might be doing it for its well-known calming effects. But beyond just sipping the liquid, the very aroma can start to soothe your nervous system. And don't get me started on the visual pleasure of watching those beautiful flowers dance in the hot water as they unfurl and release their essence. There's an artistic joy in the process, and the more you engage with it, the more you'll find that the benefits go beyond the measurable compounds in your cup.

But what about the practicalities? For instance, does the water quality matter? Absolutely! Whether you're making an infusion or a decoction, the quality of your water can have a profound impact. You're coaxing these plants to give up their essence, after all. Think of water as the carrier of these medicinal properties. So, always go for purified or spring water when possible. And while we're at it, the vessel you're using matters too. Glass or ceramic is generally best as it doesn't react with the herbs or retain flavors.

One important note—time is of the essence, literally. The longer you steep an infusion, the stronger it will be, both in flavor and potency. But if you let it sit for too long, it can become bitter or lose some of its aromatic qualities. So there's a balance to be struck. A good rule of thumb is to steep for around 5 to 10 minutes, but you can adjust according to taste and intention.

In the case of decoctions, timing becomes even more crucial. You're aiming to break down the hardy cell walls of roots, barks, or stems to liberate their medicinal compounds. So, not giving them enough time on the stove could mean you're missing out on the good stuff. However, simmering them for too long can destroy some of the more volatile components and may make the brew unpalatably strong. Again, balance is key, and a simmering period of 20 to 45 minutes is often the sweet spot.

At this point, you might be wondering: Can I make a big batch and store it? The answer varies. Infusions are best consumed fresh, but they can last in the fridge for up to 48 hours. Decoctions are a bit more forgiving and can be stored for up to a week. However, keep in mind that the longer they're stored, the more they lose their potency and vibrancy.

Alright, before we wander further down this winding herbal path, let's pause and recap for a moment. We've covered the elemental differences between infusions and decoctions, delved into the artistry and ritual of the brewing process, and explored the practical aspects of water quality, timing, and storage. That's a lot to take in, but remember, this is a journey, and you've got the best guides— your intuition and the plants themselves. As you continue to experiment, observe, and, most importantly, enjoy the process, you'll find your own unique rhythm and style.

So, ready for the next adventure in this herbal odyssey? Trust me; it only gets more exciting from here!

Techniques and Ratios

Alright, buckle up! We're about to dive into the nitty-gritty of techniques and ratios for brewing herbal infusions and decoctions. It's a world filled with as much art as science, where intuition often partners with precise measurements to create something extraordinary.

Imagine, if you will, a painter before a blank canvas. Each stroke, each color, each shade is deliberately chosen, yet the end result is often a surprise even to the artist. Similarly, brewing herbal concoctions is an interplay between careful calculation and the sheer joy of creation. You don't have to be an alchemist or a chemist to get it right, but a little understanding of techniques and ratios can go a long way.

So, let's begin with the basics: the plant-to-water ratio. Most standard infusions call for one to two tablespoons of dried herbs per cup of boiling water. Now, you might wonder, why dried herbs? Well, drying not only preserves herbs but also concentrates their medicinal compounds. However, if you have fresh herbs—plucked straight from your garden or sourced from a trustworthy supplier— you'll generally need more, as they contain more water. The rule of thumb is to use three times as much fresh herb as dried, though this could vary based on the herb's water content. For fresh herbs, a ratio of one to three tablespoons per cup of water is a good starting point.

You know how the simple act of toasting spices in a dry pan can elevate a dish? The same applies to some herbs. Gently toasting them before infusion can unlock aromatic compounds, creating a more flavorful and complex brew. However, not all herbs benefit from toasting. Herbs that have volatile oils, like mint or lemon balm, are best used as is. On the flip side, some hardy roots and barks truly shine when lightly toasted. Knowing when to toast and when not to requires a bit of practice, but it's well worth the exploration.

Let's talk water temperature. Boiling water is not universally ideal for all herbs. Delicate leaves and flowers might just need water that's been brought to a near boil, then allowed to cool for a minute or two. A slightly lower temperature can help preserve the nuanced flavors and volatile oils. Roots and barks, however, can withstand and indeed require full boiling water to break down their tough cellular structure. Again, there are no hard and fast rules, only guidelines, and your taste and needs should dictate the specifics.

What about the brewing time? Timing, as they say, is everything. In a fast-paced world, it's tempting to rush the steeping process, but patience is your friend here. A quick steep of a few minutes might give you a lovely aroma and flavor, but to truly unlock the therapeutic benefits, a longer steep time is often needed. A 15-20 minute steep is great for most infusions, but for maximum extraction of medicinal compounds, you might go up to an hour.

For decoctions, you're typically dealing with much tougher plant materials like roots, barks, and some seeds. These hardy plant parts often have their medicinal compounds locked away behind sturdy cell walls. Breaking these down requires a little more effort, usually in the form of simmering the material in water for an extended period. Twenty to 45 minutes is a good range, but as with infusions, experimentation is encouraged. Pay attention to color and aroma as indicators of when your decoction is ready.

Now, what if you want to mix things up? Literally! Combining herbs in a single infusion or decoction brings us into the realm of herbal synergy. Two or more herbs can often work together to enhance each other's beneficial effects or to balance out any harshness. But how do you know what ratios to use for each herb in a mixture? Start simple. If you're making a calming evening tea, you might blend equal parts of chamomile, lavender, and lemon balm. As you gain more experience and confidence, you can start to adjust the ratios to better suit your tastes and health needs.

There's a rich tapestry of variables that can impact the final outcome of your brew, from the quality and freshness of your herbs to the mineral content of your water. Don't be daunted. Your own senses of smell, taste, and even sight are invaluable tools in this endeavor.

If this feels like a lot, don't worry. It's a journey, not a sprint. The beauty of mastering techniques and ratios is that you become free to improvise, to play. Each cup you brew is a chance to learn and refine your skills. It's akin to learning a musical instrument; the scales and chords might feel cumbersome at first, but they're the building blocks of every beautiful melody you'll ever play.

So, let your brews be your symphonies, complex orchestrations of flavor, aroma, and wellness. With the principles of technique and ratios in your toolkit, the possibilities are as boundless as your imagination. Ready for the next deep dive? Because we're far from done exploring this amazing world of herbal infusions and decoctions.

So where were we? Ah yes, we were diving into the intricate world of herbal infusions and decoctions. Think of it like cooking—once you understand the basic techniques, the kitchen—or in this case, the teapot—becomes your oyster.

One subject we haven't yet touched on is the role of vessels and containers. It's not just about any pot, cup, or teapot. The material of the vessel can also impact the final brew. Stainless steel, glass, or ceramic pots are generally the go-to for most herbalists. They don't react with the herbs and offer a neutral base. Plastics and aluminum, on the other hand, might leach undesirable substances into your brew, altering both flavor and safety. So if you've been considering investing in that beautiful porcelain teapot, now might be the time.

And here's a pro tip: pre-warming your teapot or infusion vessel can make a difference. Pouring hot water into a cold vessel can cause a sudden drop in temperature, which may affect the brewing process. So, give your vessel a quick rinse with hot water to warm it up before adding your herbs.

Now, onto straining techniques. A fine-mesh strainer is a staple in any herbalist's toolkit. The aim is to separate the solid plant matter, leaving behind a clear liquid. But did you ever consider that the straining process itself could affect the strength of your infusion? If you press down on the herbs while straining, you might extract additional compounds, making your infusion stronger. This could be a good or a bad thing, depending on the herb and your specific health needs. Being mindful of how you strain your brew can thus be an important part of the technique.

Straining also has another dimension: particle size. The size to which the herb is cut or ground can impact how quickly its medicinal compounds are released into the water. A finely ground herb will have more surface area in contact with the water, resulting in quicker and potentially stronger brews. But beware, some herbs release bitter compounds if ground too finely and brewed for too long. It's all about finding that Goldilocks zone for each specific herb or blend.

Timing and temperature, vessel and straining, ratios and blends—they all work in harmony to create that perfect cup. And let's not forget the final, magical element: your intention. Whether it's a cup to help you relax, to relieve a specific ailment, or simply to enjoy the sheer pleasure of herbal flavors, the intention you put into the process can also be considered an essential 'ingredient'. As many traditional cultures believe, the energy and attention you give to the making of the brew can be just as therapeutic as the herbs themselves.

Then there's the marvel of tasting notes. As you refine your techniques, you'll start to notice nuanced flavors and aromas that you may have missed earlier. The first sip might bring forth the floral notes, the second sip might highlight the herb's earthiness, and the last might have a surprising hint of sweetness. All these layers of complexity aren't just there for your taste buds to enjoy; they're also indicative of the various compounds at work, providing a multi-faceted approach to well-being.

Finally, always remember to take notes. The path to mastering techniques and ratios is one of trial and error. Document your successes, and perhaps more importantly, your less-than-perfect attempts. Your future self will thank you.

So there you have it, a winding journey through the art and science of brewing herbal infusions and decoctions. The techniques are your colors, the ratios your brushstrokes, and each brew a canvas waiting for your personal touch. As you sip your next cup, take a moment to marvel at the complexity and beauty encapsulated in that simple act. It's not just leaves and water; it's a holistic experience, nurtured by knowledge, technique, and a touch of alchemy. Enjoy the brew, and most of all, enjoy the process.

Mastering the art of brewing herbal infusions and decoctions involves a careful balance of technique, ratio, and a keen understanding of your ingredients. Let's break down some of the most common methods, their unique quirks, safety protocols, and the types of herbs best suited for each.

Method 1: Simple Infusion
1. **Step-by-Step Instructions**:
    1. Boil water and let it cool for a minute.
    2. Add 1 to 2 teaspoons of dried herbs per cup of water to your teapot or jar.
    3. Pour the hot water over the herbs.
    4. Cover the vessel to keep volatile oils from escaping.
    5. Steep for 5 to 15 minutes.
    6. Strain and enjoy!
2. **Unique Quirks**: Perfect for delicate herbs like chamomile and mint. Simple and quick.
3. **Safety Protocols**: Make sure to cover the vessel to keep beneficial oils from evaporating. Always strain properly to remove all plant matter.

4. **Ideal Plant Types**: Soft leaves and flowers like chamomile, peppermint, and lemon balm.

Method 2: Cold Infusion
1. **Step-by-Step Instructions**:
    1. Add 1 to 2 teaspoons of dried herbs to a jar.
    2. Cover with cold water.
    3. Seal the jar and let it steep in the fridge for at least 4 hours or overnight.
    4. Strain and enjoy chilled or at room temperature.
2. **Unique Quirks**: Cold infusions draw out different compounds than hot methods, often resulting in a milder flavor.
3. **Safety Protocols**: Always refrigerate during steeping to prevent bacterial growth.
4. **Ideal Plant Types**: Marshmallow root, slippery elm, and chia seeds.

Method 3: Decoction
1. **Step-by-Step Instructions**:
    1. Add 1 to 2 teaspoons of dried roots or barks to a pot.
    2. Cover with cold water.
    3. Bring to a boil and simmer for 20 to 45 minutes.
    4. Strain and serve.
2. **Unique Quirks**: Great for extracting tough, woody compounds.
3. **Safety Protocols**: Boiling can evaporate volatile compounds, so keep the pot covered during simmering.
4. **Ideal Plant Types**: Woody and root-based herbs like ginger root, cinnamon bark, and dandelion root.

Method 4: Solar and Lunar Infusions
1. **Step-by-Step Instructions**:
    1. Prepare herbs and water as you would for a simple infusion.
    2. Cover the jar and place it in direct sunlight or moonlight for 4 to 6 hours.
    3. Strain and enjoy.
2. **Unique Quirks**: Adds an esoteric flair to your brew and is thought by some to enhance the energetic properties of the herbs.
3. **Safety Protocols**: Ensure the jar is properly sealed to avoid contamination.
4. **Ideal Plant Types**: Herbs with spiritual or mystical associations, like sage or mugwort.

Remember, mastering these techniques and ratios is a journey. What I've given you here are more like guidelines than strict rules. Adjust ratios, steeping times, and temperatures according to your personal preferences and health needs. Most importantly, always consult healthcare professionals when using herbs for medicinal purposes, especially if you're pregnant, nursing, or taking other medications. Happy brewing!

Popular Herbal Infusions and Their Benefits

So, you've got the techniques down, you've been playing around with ratios, and now you're staring at an herb shelf that would make even the most seasoned botanist's head spin. The question is, which herbs do you actually pick? And once you've picked them, what can they do for you?

Let me introduce you to some of the rockstars of the herbal world. These herbs not only have incredible flavors but also offer a range of health benefits that you'll be keen to explore. Let's start this chapter by shedding light on some of the most popular herbal infusions and the benefits they bring to the table, or rather, to the teacup. Trust me; this will turn your tea-drinking into a whole new kind of ritual—one that's not only pleasurable but also wonderfully beneficial for your health.

Chamomile: The comforter, the universal hug-in-a-mug! Chamomile has been loved for ages for its calming properties. Having a stressful day? Chamomile. Can't sleep? Chamomile. It's a go-to for its calming effects on the nervous system, and it's excellent for your digestive system too. You know that old saying, "When you're nervous, listen to your gut"? Well, chamomile soothes both the gut and the nerves. How neat is that?

Mint: Next up is the invigorating, the zesty, the one-and-only: mint. Talk about versatility! This herb has been a stalwart in both culinary and medicinal use. While its most straightforward application is for refreshing breath, this powerhouse does more than that. Peppermint can aid digestion and help relieve headaches. Its cooling sensation also makes it a hit for combating summer heat. Picture this: a hot summer day, you, and an ice-cold glass of peppermint infusion. Pure bliss!

Green Tea: Now, this one's a bit of an overachiever. Green tea is abundant in antioxidants and a variety of polyphenols that benefit everything from your heart health to your skin. It's like that classmate who excels in every subject and yet is incredibly humble about it. If you're looking to add a health kick to your day, green tea is your buddy.

Ginger: Okay, imagine this. You wake up, it's freezing outside, and your body feels like it's made of lead. Enter ginger, the warm hug your soul needs. Ginger is a fiery root with a bit of a kick, making it perfect for those days when you need a bit of a pick-me-up. Apart from giving you that warm feeling inside, ginger is excellent for combating nausea and aiding digestion.

Lavender: Picture yourself in a field of purple, surrounded by a mesmerizing scent—that's the power of lavender. This herb is often linked with relaxation and good sleep, but did you know it's also used for minor burns and cuts due to its antiseptic properties? It's like having a mini first-aid kit right in your garden. Just steep some lavender buds in hot water and let your worries drift away.

Turmeric: This golden spice is like the Midas of the herbal world. Its active ingredient, curcumin, has potent anti-inflammatory properties. Imagine being able to combat inflammation just by sipping a delicious, golden brew. It's almost like a superpower, isn't it?

Echinacea: This one's the warder-offer of colds. Yes, I know that's not a real word, but you get what I mean. Echinacea has been found to boost the immune system, making it a popular choice during flu season.

Rosemary: This fragrant herb is a star in the kitchen, but did you know it also improves memory and concentration? It's the scholar of the herb world, helping you focus just when you need it.

Nettle: The misunderstood nettle. Often dismissed as a pesky weed, this plant is actually a nutrient powerhouse, rich in iron and vitamin C. Perfect for when you need a little pick-me-up.

Rooibos: Originating from South Africa, this red tea is caffeine-free and rich in antioxidants. It's your chill friend who still knows how to bring the party.

Licorice Root: Sweet and soothing, licorice root is like the grandma of the herbal world—always there to make you feel better, especially when it comes to digestive issues.

Sage: With its unique peppery flavor, sage is not only a culinary gem but also a defender against inflammation. Sage advice? Include more of it in your diet!

Thyme: Beyond its culinary uses, thyme has antiviral properties that make it a wonderful addition to your winter wellness routine. Just like that reliable friend who's always got tissues and hand sanitizer.

Dandelion: Often overlooked as a weed, dandelion leaves are actually edible and filled with vitamins A, C, and K. The underdog that's secretly a superhero in your backyard!

Fennel: With a flavor reminiscent of licorice, fennel is excellent for digestion and has been known to help with everything from menstrual cramps to bloating. It's your ultimate self-care companion.

Cinnamon: This warming spice isn't just for desserts; it's also great for regulating blood sugar levels. It's like that friend who's sweet but knows when to keep you in check.

Hibiscus: Known for its vibrant color and tart flavor, hibiscus is high in vitamin C and may help lower blood pressure. It's the life of the party, bringing both fun and benefits.

Become a "Mixologist"

It's like being a mixologist, but for your garden and your well-being. So, let's get into some mix-and-match suggestions to get you brewing some delightful concoctions.

Chamomile & Lavender: This combo is like a cozy blanket for your soul. Chamomile brings in the calming vibes, and lavender complements it with a touch of aromatic relaxation. This blend is perfect for winding down after a long day.

Mint & Lemon Balm: The zing of mint with the soothing touch of lemon balm. Think of this as your afternoon pick-me-up without the caffeine. It's refreshing and invigorating, without keeping you awake at night.

Rosemary & Thyme: These two are the dynamic duo of the savory world. Their earthy flavors complement each other like a dream. Use this blend to infuse oils or to add a rich, aromatic touch to your meals.

Nettle & Ginger: Spice up your nettle tea with a slice of ginger. Nettle offers a grassy, rich flavor, while ginger adds warmth and spiciness. It's like a warm hug in a mug and a good way to give your immune system a little nudge.

Rooibos & Cinnamon: Cinnamon can add a spicy, sweet dimension to the earthy flavor of rooibos. This blend could become your go-to winter warmer or an iced delight for summer.

Basil & Oregano: These two Mediterranean favorites bring out the best in each other. Try them in tomato-based dishes, pestos, or as an infusion for an herbal twist on your cooking.

Sage & Rosemary: These two make an excellent pair for your more hearty, robust dishes. Think roasted meats or root vegetables. As a tea, they offer a powerful earthy flavor.

Echinacea & Elderberry: Both of these are known for their immune-boosting properties. Mix them together for a tincture or tea that's not just medicinal, but also surprisingly pleasant to the palate.

Calendula & Chamomile: Both are gentle and soothing, making them great for skincare. You can blend them together in an oil infusion for topical application or as a tea for gut health.

Turmeric & Black Pepper: In the health world, this pair is practically iconic. Black pepper helps your body absorb turmeric more efficiently. Add these to your cooking or blend them into a tea for an anti-inflammatory boost.

Remember, blending herbs is as much about intuition as it is about knowledge. Listen to your body and adjust your blends as you go. Always consider any potential allergies or interactions with medications you might be taking. And of course, when in doubt, less is more. You can always add more herbs, but it's not so easy to take them away once they're blended. Happy blending!

Chapter 7: Antibiotics from Nature

A chapter that seems like it's straight out of a science fiction novel—Antibiotics from Nature. Yet, it's as real as it gets, rooted in practices that have survived the test of time. While our reliance on synthetic antibiotics has skyrocketed in the modern era, the natural world has been quietly offering its own antibiotic solutions all along. Mother Nature, it seems, was the original pharmacist. In this chapter, we'll dig deep into the rich, fascinating world of natural antibiotics, tracing their origins and charting their re-emergence in a world that's starting to feel the limitations of synthetic options.

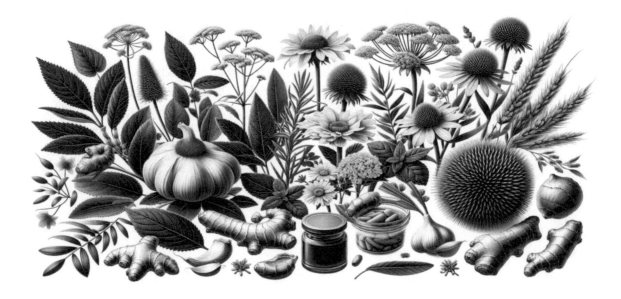

The history of antibiotics reads like a thrilling adventure, full of unexpected discoveries and urgent quests. Imagine it's 1928, and you're Alexander Fleming, who, returning to his lab after a holiday, finds a petri dish where mold has killed the surrounding bacteria. And boom! Penicillin enters the scene. But hold on, this isn't just the story of men in white coats making groundbreaking discoveries. If we trace back even further, we'll find indigenous communities using molds, plant extracts, and other natural substances to treat infections. The ancient Egyptians, for example, applied moldy bread to wounds. So, in a way, Fleming's discovery was more of a rediscovery.

Now, let's shift gears and talk about herbal alternatives to common antibiotics. Are you surprised to hear that garlic can give some synthetic antibiotics a run for their money? Or that the cute little daisies called Echinacea can stimulate your immune system? Even kitchen staples like thyme and oregano pack a punch when it comes to antibacterial properties. We'll dive deep into the how and why of these natural powerhouses, explaining how you can integrate them into your lifestyle for both preventive and curative measures.

Of course, we can't talk about antibiotics without discussing safety. The rules of engagement, so to speak, are a bit different in the herbal realm. For one, natural doesn't necessarily mean harmless. Secondly, these herbs come with their own sets of precautions and possible interactions. Don't worry, we'll guide you through it, so you're not just throwing a hodgepodge of herbs into your tea and hoping for the best.

In summary, this chapter aims to open a new window into your understanding of antibiotics—one where past meets present, and nature meets science. Here, you'll get the opportunity to become your own health advocate, responsibly and effectively making choices that align with both age-old wisdom and modern understanding. Intrigued? Good, let's start this journey together.

A Brief History of Antibiotics

The history of antibiotics! It's a tale so intriguing it could very well rival any bestselling thriller, complete with serendipitous discoveries, a race against time, and humanity's ceaseless battle against microscopic enemies. Ready to dig into this narrative? Let's get going.

Picture this: It's the dawn of human civilization, long before lab coats and sterile environments were a thing. Our ancestors are roaming the earth, living off the land, and getting into all sorts of scrapes and skirmishes. They're cutting themselves on sharp stones, getting bitten by animals, and coming down with diseases that they have no names for. And yet, they're surviving—not always, but often enough. How, you ask? Well, they're keen observers of nature, and they're picking up on its cues. They see that certain leaves or plant extracts can help accelerate wound healing or combat infections. They may not know why, but they know that it works, and that's good enough for them.

Fast-forward to the ancient civilizations—the Egyptians, Indians, and Chinese, to name a few. They are refining these practices, documenting them, and even integrating them into their spiritual and ritualistic lives. Take the ancient Egyptians, for instance. They had this practice of applying moldy bread to wounds. Unbeknownst to them, that bread was teeming with natural antibiotic agents. Similarly, in ancient China and India, botanicals like garlic and turmeric were already highly prized for their medicinal properties. Little did they know that these simple herbs were the antibiotics of their day.

As we move into medieval times, we see the wisdom of these practices carried forward, albeit interspersed with some rather quirky ideas. Leech therapy, anyone? But even then, amidst all the misconceptions, the core understanding that natural substances could combat disease persisted. Monks, who were the physicians of their time, often grew their own medicinal gardens and had an intimate understanding of herbal remedies. They might not have understood the science behind it, but their empirical evidence was strong.

Now, let's swing over to the late 19th and early 20th centuries, a period brimming with scientific curiosity and innovations. Louis Pasteur and Robert Koch are setting the stage for modern bacteriology. Pasteur's work on germ theory and Koch's discoveries of specific bacteria responsible for diseases like tuberculosis and cholera are laying the groundwork for targeted treatments. And then, of course, came the watershed moment in 1928, with Alexander Fleming and his accidental discovery of penicillin. Walking into his cluttered lab after a vacation, Fleming noticed that a mold called Penicillium notatum had killed off the surrounding bacteria in a petri dish. Eureka!

Fleming's discovery was groundbreaking, but penicillin was not mass-produced until World War II, when its life-saving potential became glaringly obvious. The antibiotic era had officially dawned. Pharmaceutical companies jumped on the bandwagon, and new antibiotics like streptomycin, tetracycline, and chloramphenicol were introduced. It was a golden age of sorts, a time when it seemed like bacterial infections would soon be a thing of the past.

However, our story takes a darker turn here, as misuse and overuse of antibiotics lead to resistant strains of bacteria. Our overreliance on these miracle drugs is proving to be our Achilles heel. Nature, it seems, is fighting back, evolving faster than we can come up with new drugs. This brings us to the current era, where there's a renewed interest in natural antibiotics and traditional practices. The stage is set for a full-circle moment, as we find ourselves revisiting the wisdom of ancient civilizations, now backed by scientific research.

As we face the challenges of antibiotic resistance, there's a growing awareness that the solutions might lie not just in futuristic labs, but also in our backyards, kitchens, and even in ancient texts gathering dust in some forgotten library. It's a humbling thought, isn't it? That despite all our technological advances, we may need to turn back to the roots, literally and metaphorically, to find sustainable ways to fight infections.

So, that's a whirlwind tour of the history of antibiotics, from primitive balms to pills and injections, and perhaps back to nature again. It's a story of triumphs, setbacks, and rediscoveries. We've come a long way, but as it turns out, the journey is far from over. With antibiotic resistance posing new challenges, could the next chapter in this gripping tale be written by someone like you, inspired to merge the old with the new in creative, effective ways? One can only hope.

As we leave behind the golden age of antibiotics and grapple with the harsh realities of antibiotic resistance, we're entering a new era—one that's pushing us to rethink our relationship with these wonder drugs. There's a resurgence of interest in alternative therapies, and this is where the field gets really fascinating. We are seeing an increasing amount of research focused on understanding the mechanisms behind natural antibiotics, as well as ways to synergize these with synthetic ones to tackle resistant bacteria. Scientists are looking at a myriad of sources—soil samples from remote locations, exotic plants, even compounds isolated from marine organisms. The message is clear: our quest for effective antibiotics is not bound by the confines of traditional labs; it's an all-encompassing, interdisciplinary effort that taps into multiple aspects of science and traditional knowledge.

Let's not forget the rise of precision medicine, a burgeoning field that aims to tailor healthcare at an individual level. With advancements in genomics and data analytics, the potential to develop highly targeted antibiotics is growing. Imagine a future where your antibiotic prescription is tailored not just to the bacterial strain you're fighting but also to your genetic makeup. It's like having a bespoke suit made, but for your health. This approach could potentially reduce side-effects and make treatment more efficient, although ethical considerations like accessibility and data privacy need to be carefully negotiated.

Interestingly, many of the advancements in synthetic antibiotics are inadvertently mirroring the wisdom found in natural alternatives. For example, antibiotic cocktails—combinations of two or more antibiotics—are now being developed to tackle resistant bacteria, echoing the holistic approach of herbal medicine, where multiple herbs are often used in tandem to treat illnesses. The synergistic effects of combining different antibiotics might just give us the upper hand in our ongoing battle against bacterial foes. And guess what? This is something herbalists have known for centuries; combining different herbs can often yield more potent remedies than using them in isolation.

However, it's not all sunshine and roses. The increased interest in natural antibiotics also brings up pressing ethical and ecological issues. As people scavenge remote landscapes for the next miracle cure, the risk of depleting precious natural resources looms large. And then there's the inevitable question of who 'owns' these natural remedies—can pharmaceutical companies patent substances that indigenous communities have been using for generations?

Which brings us back to square one—the need for a balanced, respectful, and holistic approach, one that combines the rigor of modern science with the wisdom of traditional practices. This balance could be our most potent weapon in combating the looming threat of antibiotic resistance. And this approach goes beyond just medicine; it's a philosophy that we can apply to multiple facets of our lives, from agriculture to sanitation to community health initiatives.

So, there you have it—the enthralling narrative of antibiotics, from the first accidental discoveries to the challenges and opportunities that lie ahead. It's a narrative that's still unfolding, written by scientists, researchers, traditional healers, and perhaps even by you. It serves as a poignant reminder of the intricacies of the natural world, the ingenuity of human beings, and the complexity of our ongoing relationship with the microscopic universe that lives within and around us. It's a story where the past informs the present and inspires the future, a symbiotic relationship that we would do well to nurture as we look toward the horizon of healthcare. With antibiotic resistance as one of the most urgent healthcare issues of our time, the stakes are high, but so are the opportunities for groundbreaking work in the field. Will we rise to the challenge? Given the resilience and ingenuity that have marked our journey thus far, I'd like to think so.

Herbal Alternatives to Common Antibiotics

Picture this: you're a bit under the weather, the doctor prescribes you antibiotics, and while you're waiting at the pharmacy, you ponder, "Isn't there a more natural way to do this?" Well, my friend, the answer is a resounding yes, and that's exactly what we're diving into right now. The amazing thing is, nature has already been doing what pharmaceutical companies spend billions trying to achieve. It's like nature is the OG antibiotic lab, way ahead of the curve, and we're just now catching up to see how brilliant it is.

Let's start our journey with garlic. Garlic, the staple of Italian cuisine and also one of the oldest known medicinal plants. You could say garlic is like the elder statesman of herbal antibiotics. Allicin, its active compound, is a potent antimicrobial agent. Even Louis Pasteur, the father of modern medicine, was fascinated by its antibiotic properties. And what's fascinating is that garlic's potency is activated through a unique ritual—crushing or chopping it activates its enzymatic processes, releasing allicin. It's as if the plant is telling us, "Hey, work a bit to unlock my full potential!"

But let's not stop at garlic; we have an entire botanical arsenal to explore. Echinacea is another heavy hitter in this league. Native to North America, this plant was originally used by the indigenous communities for various ailments, including infections. Modern studies back this up, showing its effectiveness in fighting respiratory infections and boosting the immune system. It's like the encouraging coach on your wellness journey, not doing the hard work for you, but certainly making the process easier.

As we discuss plant-based antibiotics, how can we forget the evergreen tea tree? Native to Australia, tea tree oil is a powerhouse with its antimicrobial and antifungal properties. However, unlike many antibiotics that act like a sledgehammer, destroying both good and bad bacteria, tea tree oil is more discerning. Think of it as a skilled archer, aiming precisely at the pathogens while sparing your beneficial gut bacteria. A word to the wise, though: its potency also means you have to handle it carefully. It should never be ingested and must always be diluted before topical application.

Ginger is another plant that deserves a special mention. Often considered a universal medicine in Ayurveda, ginger has an array of compounds like gingerol that have antibacterial properties. It's like that friend who's good at everything—whether you're dealing with nausea or a sore throat, ginger is there to lend a helping hand. But it's not just a jack-of-all-trades; research shows that it can even inhibit the growth of bacteria that are resistant to standard antibiotics. Now, that's impressive!

As we dig deeper into the world of plant-based antibiotics, we encounter the lesser-known but equally formidable goldenseal. With its roots in Native American medicine, goldenseal has berberine, a compound that fights bacteria and fungi. Picture berberine as that behind-the-scenes movie director who orchestrates the entire show but rarely gets front-page credits. Berberine increases the efficacy of the immune system by stimulating the production of white blood cells, the body's natural defense mechanism.

Now, let's switch gears and talk about the intersection of herbal and conventional medicine. The synergy between herbal alternatives and pharmaceutical antibiotics offers an intriguing possibility. Researchers are beginning to look at how herbal medicines can work alongside antibiotics to boost their effectiveness or reduce resistance. For instance, some herbs can act as "resistance modulators," which essentially means they make bacteria more susceptible to antibiotics. It's like having a wingman who makes you look good, amplifying your strengths and minimizing your weaknesses.

But we should tread carefully. While herbal antibiotics hold great promise, self-prescribing them without proper knowledge can do more harm than good. These are not one-size-fits-all solutions and their efficacy can vary depending on multiple factors like your individual constitution, the nature of the infection, and even the soil in which the plant was grown. It's crucial to consult healthcare professionals, ideally those trained in both herbal and conventional medicine, for a more holistic and personalized treatment plan.

We must also consider the environmental impact of the growing demand for these herbs. Sustainable and ethical harvesting is not just a buzzword; it's a necessity. If we're raiding Mother Nature's pharmacy at an unsustainable rate, we risk depleting these valuable resources, potentially driving some species to extinction. So, let's remember to give back to nature as much as we take.

As we wrap up this long but hopefully enlightening chat, let's ponder the potential in combining the cutting-edge techniques of modern medicine with the time-tested remedies of herbal medicine. It's a dialogue between the old and the new, tradition and innovation, a dialogue that could hold the answers to some of our most pressing healthcare challenges. So, the next time you find yourself reaching for that antibiotic pill, maybe take a moment to consider the natural alternatives that have stood the test of time. Who knows? The solution to our antibiotic crisis might just be growing in your own backyard.

As we venture further into the realm of plant-based antibiotics, another player you'll want to meet is oregano. Yes, the same oregano you sprinkle generously over your pizza also has powerful antibiotic properties. Carvacrol, the active compound in oregano, gives this herb its antibacterial punch. It's like that surprise guest at a party who turns out to be the life of the event—unassuming at first, but absolutely unforgettable once you get to know it. Research has shown that carvacrol is effective against various bacteria, including E. coli and Salmonella. This gives oregano oil its reputation as a natural antibiotic and antifungal agent. Imagine a kitchen herb doubling as a medicinal powerhouse—that's oregano for you.

Another surprising yet powerful natural antibiotic is honey. Yes, that same sticky, sweet stuff you drizzle on your pancakes or mix with your tea. Beyond its culinary uses, honey has a rich medicinal history. It's like the renaissance person of natural remedies, proficient in multiple skills—antibacterial, antifungal, and even antiviral. The magic here lies in its composition. It has a low pH and high sugar concentration, which makes it hostile for bacteria. Plus, it contains hydrogen peroxide, a known antiseptic. It's a bit like a superhero with multiple powers, each contributing to its ultimate goal: keeping infections at bay. Manuka honey from New Zealand has even been studied for its potent antibacterial properties and is currently being considered for treating antibiotic-resistant infections.

So, you're probably asking, "This all sounds great, but how do I go about using these herbal antibiotics?" Well, each herb has its own set of guidelines. For example, garlic is best consumed raw to preserve its allicin content. Oregano oil should be diluted before use, and honey should not be given to infants under one year due to the risk of botulism. It's like each plant has its own user manual, so to speak. Reading and understanding this manual is crucial to making the most of their antibiotic properties while also ensuring safety.

And speaking of safety, while these herbal alternatives are exciting and promising, they are not a direct replacement for pharmaceutical antibiotics in every case. There's a growing body of research that aims to understand the complexities of these herbal remedies better. So, think of them as complementary to traditional medicine rather than a complete substitute. The key here is to consult a healthcare professional, particularly one well-versed in herbal medicine, to determine what's best for you. You wouldn't want to dive into the deep end without learning how to swim first, right?

Another crucial consideration is drug interactions. While plants have been used safely for thousands of years, combining them with modern medication without proper guidance can be risky. For example, garlic and ginger are blood thinners and can interact with anticoagulant medications. It's a bit like mixing drinks; some combinations are delightful, while others can leave you with a terrible hangover.

As the conversation around antibiotic resistance continues to gain momentum, the role of herbal alternatives becomes even more significant. We're in a space where collaborative research between modern and traditional medicine can offer groundbreaking solutions. It's like two different schools of thought coming together for a common cause. While this collaboration promises a holistic approach to health and wellness, it also emphasizes the importance of responsible use of both herbal and pharmaceutical antibiotics. After all, too much of a good thing is never good, whether we're talking about synthetic drugs or natural herbs.

So, as we continue to explore the world of natural antibiotics, remember that this journey is about coexistence rather than replacement. It's not about turning your back on modern medicine but embracing a more holistic approach that considers the best of both worlds. And who knows? This synergy could be the key to unlocking a future where antibiotics are used more sustainably, effectively, and harmoniously with nature's bounty.

Chapter 8: Harvesting and Drying Your Herbs

This chapter is like the grand finale after the diligent work you've put into cultivating your herbal garden. You see, there's something truly magical about the first harvest. It's the moment when you can finally revel in the fruits—or rather, leaves and roots—of your labor. And, let's not forget the sweet, earthy aroma that fills the air when you snip those first sprigs of rosemary or clip those aromatic lavender buds.

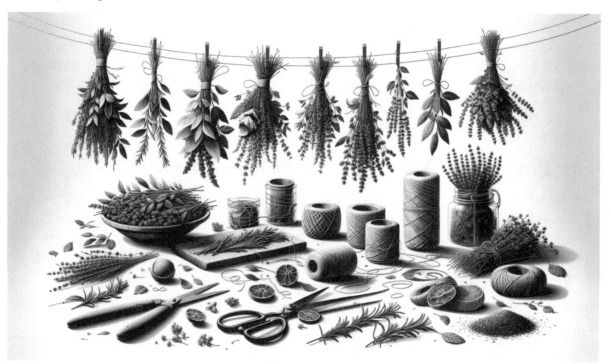

Now, it's not just about hacking away at your herb garden willy-nilly. Harvesting is an art, my friends, a dance between you and the plants that have been your green companions for so long. First up, timing is everything. Picture this: It's early morning, the dew has settled lightly on the leaves, and the world seems fresh and new. This is the perfect time to harvest most herbs. Why? Because the essential oils in herbs are at their peak during the cool, early hours, and you want to capture that goodness. That's not a hard and fast rule for every single herb, but it's a good general practice.

Now, let's talk about the how. Snips, scissors, or shears—what's your weapon of choice? In general, it's best to use sharp, clean cutting tools to make precise, clean cuts. This isn't just about aesthetics; it helps the plant heal faster too. There's also the angle of the cut, the height from the ground—oh, so many little details, but they all contribute to either the flourishing or floundering of your herbs. For example, if you're harvesting basil, make your cut just above a pair of leaves, encouraging more leafy growth.

As for drying, oh, where do we begin? Hanging bunches of herbs in a dark, well-ventilated area is the classic go-to method, a timeless picture right out of a rustic, country kitchen. But, hey, we're in modern times, and there are other ways too. Oven drying, for instance, is great for when you're in a pinch—pun intended. Dehydrators offer the advantage of controlled, consistent heat, providing excellent results, especially for moisture-rich herbs. But here's the kicker: each method has its own quirks, like the optimum temperature and duration to preserve the herbs' colors and flavors.

And finally, let's not neglect the last stage—storing those precious dried herbs. Glass jars with airtight lids are a popular choice, as they protect the herbs from moisture and light, two things that could compromise their quality. Proper labeling is also crucial. You don't want to mistake your oregano for your parsley when you're in the middle of cooking a romantic Italian dinner, now, do you?

So, there you have it, the ins and outs, the dos and don'ts of harvesting and drying your herbs. This chapter will delve into these topics with the depth and detail they deserve, so roll up those sleeves, grab your shears, and let's get to it. Shall we?

Best Times and Methods for Harvesting

When you set out to harvest your herbs, you're not just grabbing a pair of scissors and snipping away. You're stepping into a long-held ritual, one that's deeply rooted in the wisdom of ages. And it all begins with understanding when to harvest, which isn't just a matter of convenience but also a question of potency, flavor, and medicinal benefits. You know how they say timing is everything? Well, when it comes to harvesting herbs, they're not kidding.

Let's consider the seasons first. Spring and summer are generally the high times for harvesting leaves and flowers. This is when your herbs are brimming with life, as the sun's energy is channeled into leaves and blossoms. When you snip a mint leaf or a chamomile flower during this period, you're capturing the essence of the plant in its prime. In contrast, roots like turmeric and ginger are best harvested in the fall or winter when the plant's energy is drawn downwards. Picture the plant hunkering down for the colder months, storing its energy in its roots. That's the power you'll tap into when you harvest roots during this period.

However, seasons are just the tip of the iceberg. Even within these broader timeframes, there's a particular moment when each plant is at its peak. And that, my dear herbal enthusiasts, is often decided by the stage of the plant's life cycle. For example, many perennial herbs are best harvested just before flowering. At this point, the plant is mature but not yet shifting its focus towards producing seeds. Imagine it as a wise elder, at the peak of knowledge and experience but not yet in retirement. This is when you'll find the highest concentration of essential oils and other beneficial compounds. Herbs like basil, sage, and rosemary are prime candidates for this kind of timing.

Daytime also plays a crucial role. Have you ever walked through a garden in the early morning? There's a certain stillness in the air, an almost sacred quality. Well, that's not just poetic—it's also practical. The early morning, after the dew has dried but before the heat of the day, is often the best time for harvesting most herbs. In these tranquil hours, the plant's oils are at their peak concentration, offering the strongest flavor and medicinal benefits. It's like catching someone at their best mood, first thing in the morning, ready to greet the world but not yet bogged down by the day's worries.

Of course, there are exceptions to every rule. For instance, some desert plants like sagebrush are more suited for afternoon harvesting when their volatile oils have warmed and activated. Think of them as night owls as opposed to morning people; their peak performance occurs a bit later in the day.

Weather also impacts your timing. A period of dry weather before harvesting can be beneficial, as too much water can dilute the plant's essential oils. On the flip side, after a solid period of rain, your roots will be plumper and easier to dig up. It's like choosing the perfect day to go to the beach; you watch the weather patterns and make your move when the conditions are just right.

You also have to consider the plant's resilience after the harvest. You don't want to take too much and weaken the plant, diminishing its chances for future growth. For annuals, this isn't much of a concern because they complete their life cycle in one season. But for perennials and biennials, it's best to take no more than a third of the plant at a time, ensuring it has enough energy to recover and flourish.

You know, when you take a step back, you realize that harvesting isn't just a task on a to-do list; it's an intimate interaction with the natural world. You're entering into a dialogue with the plants, asking them when they're ready to offer their gifts and how much they can spare. It's a beautiful dance of give and take, one that's been performed for millennia. And now, it's your turn to join in. So, the next time you stand in your garden, shears in hand, pause for a moment and tune into the rhythms of the plants, the seasons, and the very Earth itself. Trust me, it'll make all the difference.

Alright, let's dive into the methods for harvesting herbs, which is akin to choosing the right utensils for a special dinner. You wouldn't slice bread with a butter knife, right? The same principle applies to harvesting herbs. Each plant calls for specific tools and techniques to ensure that you collect it in the most effective and respectful manner. But we're not just talking about the nuts and bolts; we're delving into a sort of choreography with the natural world.

First off, let's talk about the simplest and most common method: hand-picking. This age-old technique is perfect for delicate herbs like basil, mint, and parsley. With a gentle twist and pull, you can easily remove leaves or whole stems from the plant. Now, you might be wondering, "Why the twist?" Well, by gently twisting as you pull, you're encouraging the plant to produce more growth nodes, ensuring a more bountiful harvest down the line. It's like giving your plant a little pep talk, telling it, "You can do even better!"

Then there's snipping or cutting, a method reserved for herbs with sturdier stems, such as rosemary, sage, or thyme. For this, a good pair of garden shears is your best friend. Trust me, your scissors from the kitchen drawer won't cut it—pun intended! Garden shears offer the precision and power needed to navigate through tough, woody stems without causing undue damage to the plant. The trick here is to make clean, sharp cuts to minimize the wound and expedite the healing process. It's the same reason surgeons use sharp scalpels; a clean cut is simply easier to recover from.

Now, if you're venturing into root harvesting, you're stepping into a slightly different ball game. Digging up roots requires more heavy-duty tools like a hand trowel or even a shovel for larger plants. Imagine you're a treasure hunter, armed with a map and a trusty spade, except here, the treasure is right under your feet, waiting to be unearthed. As you dig, be mindful of the root structure. Some plants have deep taproots that go straight down, like a carrot, while others have a more complex network of roots that spread outwards. You don't want to just dig in willy-nilly and risk damaging this underground architecture. Gently loosen the soil around the root first, then carefully lift it out, preserving as much of the root as possible. It's like archaeology, every move deliberate and calculated to minimize harm.

When it comes to bark and resins, the process becomes even more specialized. You might need a sharp knife to make incisions in the bark without harming the cambium layer beneath it. For resins, it's often a matter of making small cuts in the plant from which the sticky substance will ooze and harden, ready for collection. This is not for the faint of heart or the shaky of hand; you're almost performing surgery on the plant, so precision is key.

While tools are important, your hands are the most irreplaceable tools you have. You have to gauge the firmness of your grip and the angle of your cut. For instance, if you're dealing with herbs that bruise easily, a gentle touch is a must. You can't manhandle mint or basil leaves as if you're kneading dough; they require a soft, almost caressing touch to prevent bruising and loss of essential oils. Your hands need to adapt to the texture, density, and delicacy of each plant, almost like they're having a conversation without words, sensing the plant's needs and responding in kind.

Don't forget about safety protocols. Always make sure your tools are clean and sharp. Dirty or dull tools can introduce pathogens into the plant, making it susceptible to diseases. Imagine going to the doctor only to find out they're using rusty or dirty surgical tools. Not a pretty picture, is it? The same goes for plants; they deserve the same level of care and respect.

Oh, and for those of you keen on sustainability, how about creating a natural disinfectant for your tools? A mixture of tea tree oil and water can do wonders in keeping your tools sanitized without harming the environment. It's like making your own cleaning product, one that aligns with the very ethos of herbalism.

Herb types play a role too. Some herbs are fussier than others when it comes to harvesting. Take lavender, for example. This herb prefers to be harvested with longer stems, allowing you to create those picturesque lavender bunches we all adore. On the other hand, basil is less particular; you can pinch it right off and it'll just keep on growing, like that friend who's perpetually optimistic, no matter what life throws their way.

In summary, harvesting is not a one-size-fits-all kind of deal. Each plant, with its unique personality, calls for a tailored approach. From the tools you use to the time of day you step into your garden, every little detail contributes to the richness and efficacy of your herbal harvest. This is not just agriculture; it's culture in the richest sense, a tradition that bridges ancient wisdom with modern understanding. So the next time you're in your garden, feel the weight of history in your hands and the pulse of life in each plant, and know that you're part of something much larger than yourself.

Here's a simplified summary to help you quickly grasp the best times and methods for harvesting various types of herbs:

Best Times for Harvesting
1. **Morning Harvest**
   - Ideal for most herbs
   - After dew dries but before the sun gets too hot
   - Essential oils are most concentrated
2. **Midday Harvest**
   - Good for herbs with sturdy leaves or thick stems
   - Essential oils are still quite potent
3. **Evening Harvest**
   - Suitable for root crops
   - Soil is softer, easier for digging
4. **Seasonal Timing**
   - Spring: Young leaves and shoots
   - Summer: Flowers and mature leaves
   - Fall: Seeds and roots

Methods for Harvesting
1. **Hand-Picking**
   - Ideal for: Basil, Mint, Parsley
   - Quirk: Gentle twist and pull technique
   - Safety: Clean hands to prevent contamination
2. **Snipping or Cutting**
   - Ideal for: Rosemary, Sage, Thyme
   - Quirk: Sharp, clean cuts
   - Safety: Use sanitized, sharp garden shears
3. **Root Harvesting**
   - Ideal for: Dandelion, Ginseng
   - Quirk: Loosen soil first, then lift root
   - Safety: Use a clean hand trowel or shovel
4. **Bark and Resins**
   - Ideal for: Pine, Frankincense
   - Quirk: Precision incisions, avoid harming cambium layer
   - Safety: Use a sanitized, sharp knife
5. **General Handling**
   - Ideal for: All herbs

- Quirk: Adapt grip based on plant's delicacy
- Safety: Always use clean and appropriate tools

This scheme offers a snapshot, giving you a quicker, easier way to remember the important aspects of harvesting herbs. Happy harvesting!

Drying Techniques

Now comes the equally rewarding part: drying your herbs to lock in their goodness for future use. The drying process is like the "post-production" in the movie of your herbal journey, where all the raw elements are finely tuned and prepped for the big screen—or in this case, your tea cup, spice jar, or medicine cabinet.

Firstly, let's talk about the essential need for drying herbs. You see, water is life for plants, but it's also the catalyst for decay. The natural moisture within the herbs is a playground for bacteria and mold. Therefore, drying your herbs not only prolongs their shelf life but also concentrates their essential oils, making them more potent.

Now, onto the juicy details—how to dry your precious plants. And let me tell you, there's more than one way to dry a herb!

Air Drying: The Old-School Way

Air drying is the simplest and most straightforward technique, and it's been done for centuries. If you can imagine your grandma hanging bundles of lavender or sage upside down in her kitchen, you've got the picture. This method is superb for herbs that don't hold a high moisture content—think rosemary, thyme, and oregano. The process is pretty straightforward:

1. Bundle your herbs, but not too tightly.

2. Hang them in a warm, airy place.

3. Check back in about two weeks or until they crumble easily between your fingers.

Some pros and cons for you. The upside? It's natural, requires no special equipment, and it looks pretty! The downside? It can take some time, and you've got to ensure a dry environment to prevent mold.

Oven Drying: Fast and Furious

This method is great for those who can't wait to get their hands on dried herbs. And let's be honest, patience isn't everyone's strong suit. Oven drying is pretty much what it sounds like—drying herbs in your oven. This technique works well for herbs like basil, mint, and tarragon, which have higher water content and are prone to molding when air-dried. Here's the step-by-step:

1. Set your oven to the lowest possible temperature—ideally, between 100 to 135°F (35-57°C).

2. Place your herbs on an oven-safe rack for good air circulation.

3. Leave the oven door slightly ajar to allow moisture to escape.

It can take anywhere from 30 minutes to a couple of hours. Check them often; you don't want to roast them!

Food Dehydrators: The Modern Marvel

If you're a tech-savvy herbal enthusiast, this one's for you. Food dehydrators give you full control over temperature and time, making it easier to ensure the best quality. They're perfect for large batches and a wider variety of herbs, from chamomile flowers to ginseng root.

1. Spread the herbs in a single layer on the dehydrator trays.

2. Set the temperature (usually around 95-115°F or 35-46°C).

3. Set the timer, and let the machine do its magic.

Now, food dehydrators can be a bit noisy, sort of like a white noise machine. But think of it as the sound of efficiency.

Microwave Drying: For the Truly Impatient

Yes, you read that right. You can use your microwave to dry herbs. It's the fastest method, taking just minutes, but it requires careful attention. This method is great for small batches and quick experiments but be cautious—overdoing it can lead to scorched herbs. Here's how you go about it:

1. Place herbs between two paper towels.

2. Set the microwave to a low-power setting.

3. Heat in bursts of 20-30 seconds, checking in between.

Be careful though; this method is not for the faint of heart or those who wander off easily. You need to babysit the process to avoid fiery disasters. Also, this isn't ideal for all herbs, so do some research first.

Solar Drying: Harness the Power of the Sun

If you're eco-conscious or just plain love the idea of using the sun's energy, solar drying might be up your alley. This is a method that is, of course, weather-dependent. It's the midway point between air drying and using electricity-dependent methods. To go about this, you might want to use a solar dryer, which is basically a glass-covered box that utilizes the sun to heat up and circulate air. Here's a simple guide:

1. Place herbs in a thin layer inside the solar dryer.

2. Set it up in a sunny, dry location.

3. Check the herbs daily for dryness and to ensure no critters have found their way into your stash.

Solar drying takes more attention to detail and environmental factors but has the bonus of being energy-efficient and a bit faster than air-drying. Just don't attempt this on a cloudy or humid day; Mother Nature won't be doing you any favors in that scenario.

Freeze Drying: The Futuristic Way

Freeze drying is one of the most effective ways to preserve the essence and nutrients in herbs. However, it's not your run-of-the-mill household method unless you have a freeze dryer, which is not the most common kitchen gadget. But oh, it's marvelous. Freeze-drying basically involves freezing the herb and then using a high-powered vacuum to remove the ice—not just the water, but the ice—making it extremely dry and excellent for long-term storage.

1. Place herbs in a freeze-dryer chamber.

2. Let the machine freeze the herbs to extremely low temperatures.

3. The machine will gradually warm up, allowing the ice to sublimate, leaving you with incredibly dry herbs.

If you've got the coin for a freeze dryer and are serious about preserving the natural goodness of your herbs, this is the way to go.

Silica Gel Method: For the Delicate Flowers

Some herbs, especially blossoms, are delicate and lose their shape and color when dried using conventional methods. Enter silica gel—the tiny packets you find in new shoes and bags that you're NOT supposed to eat. Silica gel is a desiccant, meaning it sucks up moisture like a thirsty camel.

1. Fill a container with an inch layer of silica gel.

2. Place your herbs or blossoms gently on top.

3. Seal the container and leave it for about a week.

This method maintains the herb's original form and color, making it ideal for herbs you want to display or use in crafts, in addition to culinary or medicinal uses.

Smoking: An Age-Old Tradition

This one's more specialized but worth mentioning. Smoking herbs isn't just for meats and cheeses; it can also effectively dry and infuse herbs with a unique flavor. This method is particularly popular for culinary herbs like rosemary, sage, and oregano. Just hang your herbs over a slow-burning fire and let the smoke do its thing. Of course, you want to do this in a controlled and safe environment—no forest fires, please!

Whichever method you choose depends on your needs, the types of herbs you're drying, and the resources you have at hand. The ultimate goal is to remove moisture while preserving the herb's essential oils, which hold the flavor and medicinal properties. So, put on your herbalist hat and start experimenting with these drying techniques to discover which one, or ones, best suit your herbal endeavors.

The Right Time to Dry

One thing we haven't touched on is when to harvest and dry your herbs. Timing is crucial, you see. For most leafy herbs, the optimal time is just before they flower. This is the point where they've stored up plenty of essential oils, making them more potent. Roots, on the other hand, are generally best harvested in the fall when the plant's energy has moved downward.

And let's not forget about safety protocols. No matter the method, cleanliness is crucial. Always ensure that your herbs are free from pesticides and pollutants. Make sure your drying racks, oven trays, or any other equipment you're using are clean. Mold is not a seasoning, folks!

In the grand tapestry of herbal lore, drying your herbs is a key thread. The method you choose will depend on various factors, like your patience level, your budget, and the types of herbs you're working with. It's an art and a science, combining ancient wisdom with modern technology. And while drying herbs might seem like a small step, it's a crucial part of the journey from seed to cup, from garden to medicine cabinet. So as you dry your herbs, think of yourself not just as a gardener, but as a custodian of a time-honored tradition that has been passed down through generations. Enjoy the process, and here's to herbs that last!

Storing Dried Herbs

So, you've spent your sweet time and effort harvesting and drying your precious herbs, and you're now staring at jars full of aromatic bliss. What's the next step? Storing them—arguably one of the most crucial stages in the herbal journey. You could have the best-grown, most expertly dried herbs in the world, but if you store them poorly, well, all your work might just go to waste.

Storing herbs is a bit like putting money in a savings account; you want to maximize interest (in this case, flavor or medicinal properties) and minimize loss (decay and spoilage). When you think about storing your herbs, you're not just shoving leaves into jars. You're creating an environment where the herbs' flavors, colors, and medicinal qualities can be preserved for the long haul.

Glass jars are often the go-to for most people. Why? Glass doesn't hold onto odors, it's relatively easy to sterilize, and you can see what's inside without having to open the lid. Mason jars have that cozy, down-to-earth vibe and are also efficient for sealing in freshness. When you use glass jars, make sure they've been sterilized—either run them through a dishwasher cycle or boil them in water for 10 minutes. The lids should be airtight; no one wants stale basil or faded chamomile.

Plastic bags or containers may seem convenient, but they can be detrimental to the quality of your herbs. Plastic can harbor smells, and it's not the best for keeping moisture out. If you must use plastic, opt for food-grade, vacuum-sealed bags. These are particularly useful if you're dealing with a large volume of herbs and need to keep them fresh for as long as possible.

Once you've chosen your containers, think about where to store them. Sunlight is not an ally in this situation; it will degrade your herbs faster than you can say 'lavender.' So pick a place that's dark, cool, and dry. You might opt for a cupboard that's far away from your stove or other heat sources. Some people even go to the extent of keeping their most prized herbs in a wine cellar, which is designed to keep its contents in optimal conditions. Think of it as the VIP lounge for your herbs.

The humidity of your storage area is also something to watch out for. Too much moisture in the air can lead to moldy, spoiled herbs. You can use silica packets (the same kind used in shoe boxes) to help control moisture. Just place one in each jar, and it will absorb any excess moisture, leaving your herbs nice and dry.

Speaking of moisture, let's talk about freezer storage. Some herbs retain their flavor and medicinal properties better when stored in the freezer. The cold temperature puts them into a kind of suspended animation, preserving their life force for later use. But remember, not all herbs freeze well. Leafy herbs like basil and mint can get pretty soggy when thawed. Root herbs and barks, on the other hand, freeze beautifully.

Labeling is the unsung hero of effective herb storage. The last thing you want is to mix up your sage with your thyme when you're in the middle of a recipe—or worse, a home remedy. Always label your jars with the name of the herb and the date it was harvested or dried. Trust me, you might think you'll remember, but all dried herbs start to look alike after a while.

Now, how long can you expect your herbs to stay good? Most dried herbs have a shelf-life of one to three years, depending on the herb and the conditions in which they're stored. Over time, the oils that give herbs their flavor and medicinal properties will degrade. So it's a good idea to smell and perhaps even taste a small bit of an herb if it has been stored for a while before using it for cooking or remedies.

Safety can't be stressed enough when it comes to storing herbs, especially those used for medicinal purposes. Child-proof containers are a must if you have little ones running around. Also, separate your toxic or potentially harmful herbs from those that are safe to consume. Label them clearly and, if possible, lock them away. You're building a natural medicine cabinet, not a hazard zone.

Imagine, if you will, that you're not just an herbal enthusiast but an alchemist. Each jar in your herbal storage is like a vessel of potential, holding remedies, flavors, and fragrances that can transform simple meals into feasts, ailments into comforts, and a house into a home. The care you invest in storing your herbs pays you back in full, not just in longevity but also in the potency and effectiveness of every leaf, root, and flower you've so lovingly preserved. So the next time you unscrew the lid of a mason jar filled with dried lavender or rosemary, take a deep breath and savor not just the aroma but the tradition, foresight, and wisdom contained within.

In the realm of herb storage, rotation is another principle to keep in mind. Much like you would rotate food in your pantry to use older items first, you should do the same with your herbs. Bring the older jars to the front and put the newly harvested or dried herbs at the back. This practice ensures that you're using your herbs while they're still potent, instead of discovering a three-year-old jar of oregano that has lost much of its magic. This is especially critical for herbs that have strong medicinal properties. Their effectiveness can wane with time, and in some cases, they may even undergo chemical changes that render them less safe to use.

The power of technology! In today's modern world, tech gadgets have even found their way into the serene environment of herbal care. For the particularly dedicated, there are hygrometers, little devices that measure the level of humidity in your storage area. They're usually used for cigar storage but work well for herbs too. If the humidity levels begin to rise, you can take corrective action before your herbs are affected. Another interesting addition is vacuum sealers designed specifically for jars. These handy devices suck out all the air, giving your herbs a longer shelf-life.

There's also something to be said about the aesthetic joy of seeing your herbs neatly lined up, their varied hues and textures showcased like jewels in a treasure chest. For those who have invested in transparent jars, consider crafting little curtains or shades to place over them, adding a bit of whimsy while protecting them from light. Or, if you're into interior design, why not turn your herbal storage into a feature wall? Picture a rustic wooden shelf holding rows of mason jars filled with vibrant herbs, each labeled in beautiful calligraphy. Not only does it serve a functional purpose, but it also becomes a conversation starter, making your herbal journey a shared experience with anyone who visits your home.

Let's not forget about the importance of backup. In the world of computing, they say that data doesn't exist unless it's backed up in three different locations. While you don't need to be that rigorous with your herbs, it's not a bad idea to have a backup stash. Keep a small amount of essential herbs in a separate location. In case something unfortunate happens—say, a jar breaks, or a batch of herbs goes moldy—you won't be left scrambling.

So, you see, storing dried herbs is not just about finding a convenient spot in your kitchen cabinet. It's about creating an optimal environment that prolongs the life and preserves the quality of your cherished plants. It's about employing smart tactics to keep everything organized and within easy reach. It's about embracing technology that can give your herbs an edge in longevity. And beyond these practicalities, it's about respecting the very essence of each plant, treating them not as mere commodities but as living entities that deserve care even in their dried form.

Your herbs are your allies, whether in cooking, healing, or simply bringing aromatic joy. They deserve the same care and attention that they have given you. So the next time you find yourself in the tranquil ritual of sealing a jar of freshly dried herbs, remember that you're not just storing plants—you're safeguarding a tradition, a slice of nature, and a source of well-being for days to come.

Chapter 9: Real-Life Applications and Case Studies

We've arrived at Chapter 9, a chapter close to my heart and likely to be dear to yours as well. You see, theory and practice dance a delicate tango in the world of herbal medicine. We've explored the 'how-tos,' dived into the intricacies of crafting oils, tinctures, and infusions, and mulled over the scientific aspects. Yet, if there's one chapter that pulls it all together, making the herbal world truly relatable, it's this one—Real-Life Applications and Case Studies.

Imagine sitting around a campfire, sharing stories of how a simple chamomile tea eased a restless night, or how a tincture made from Echinacea nipped that nasty cold in the bud. Those personal experiences are the lifeblood of herbal medicine, making the green leaves, intricate roots, and vibrant petals more than just parts of a plant. They become characters in our life stories, allies in our quests for better health and well-being.

And don't worry, we're not setting sail without a compass here. As much as anecdotal tales bring color and context to the practice of using herbs, we'll also tether ourselves to the scientific rigors of clinical insights. What does the research say about the herbs you're using? How do certain plant compounds interact with human physiology on a cellular level? Is there empirical evidence that supports the centuries-old wisdom about an herb's power to heal or soothe?

When you're navigating the herbal landscape, it's easy to get lost in the foliage—each leaf of knowledge leading to a branching path of understanding. But stories bring us back to the trailhead, the human experience, reminding us that, while herbs grow in the ground, their true home is in the daily lives of people like you and me. Those who have felt their potent touch in some tangible, beautiful way. Each story, whether whispered through generational wisdom or dissected in a lab, becomes another star in the constellation of herbal knowledge.

This chapter, rich in both personal experiences and scrutinized research, aims to be that bridge between the empirically tested and the emotionally felt. It serves as a testament to the versatility and efficacy of herbal medicine in contemporary life, painting a picture that is both as old as human history and as fresh as the latest scientific paper. So, grab a cup of your favorite herbal infusion, find a cozy spot, and let's dive into the real-life applications and scientific examinations that make herbal medicine the deeply embedded practice it is today.

Personal Experiences with Herbal Medicine

There's something incredibly intimate and profound about sharing personal experiences, isn't there? Our own journeys through the maze of herbal medicine are like footprints on a dewy morning—

each step revealing a unique imprint, a story to tell. As Simon Jr. Jackson, allow me to pull back the curtain on my own history with herbal remedies, an expedition that goes beyond mere fascination or intellectual curiosity. We're talking about life-changing moments, woven together through herbs and their remarkable capabilities.

Let me start with my childhood, a time where pharmaceuticals weren't our go-to answer for every ache or cough. My mother, a fantastic gardener and healer in her own right, had an answer for almost anything in the green arms of her garden. Whenever I'd suffer from a sore throat, she would pick sage leaves and steep them into a tea. That earthy, aromatic brew worked like magic, not just easing the physical discomfort but also providing a sense of warmth and well-being that no cough syrup could ever replicate.

Fast forward to my teenage years, a time of stress, hormonal upheaval, and sleepless nights cramming for exams. Rather than reaching for over-the-counter sleep aids or anxiety meds, my introduction to lavender came at the perfect moment. A few drops of lavender essential oil on my pillowcase became a nightly ritual. And I kid you not; it was as if someone had flipped the 'calm' switch in my brain. Just the act of laying my head down became an invitation for relaxation, a segue into restful sleep that seemed to kiss my worries away.

My interest in herbal medicine started to take on a more serious tone when I entered university. Armed with the wisdom from my family and a zeal to explore more, I dove headlong into botany and natural medicine courses. This was where I met ginseng, a remarkable root that had a reputation among traditional Chinese healers for its ability to combat fatigue and enhance cognitive functions. You see, student life can be a whirlwind of lectures, part-time jobs, and social commitments. Ginseng became my herbal wingman, a secret sauce that helped me juggle these responsibilities while keeping burnout at bay.

As I ventured into adulthood, I realized that herbal medicine isn't just about individual experiences; it becomes part of a community, a shared dialogue about well-being and proactive health choices. I started cultivating my own herb garden, focusing on local plants with healing properties. I even led workshops, teaching folks how to make their own tinctures and infusions. This is when I met Susan, a woman who had suffered from chronic migraines for years. Over-the-counter medications had offered little relief, and the side effects often left her drained. Skeptical but desperate, she decided to give feverfew, a traditional remedy for migraines, a try. The change was not instantaneous but noticeable over a couple of months. Susan reported fewer migraine episodes, and when they did occur, the intensity was much less debilitating. Seeing her transformation felt like watching a seed sprout into a full-grown plant, another affirmation of herbal medicine's life-changing potential.

The landscape of herbal medicine is like an ecosystem, where each plant, each story, and each experience contributes to a larger understanding of health and wellness. From treating minor ailments to managing chronic conditions, the arsenal of herbs has proven time and again to be both versatile and effective. It's not just about the past, ancient recipes handed down through generations. It's about the present moment, where modern research and age-old wisdom can cross-pollinate, enhancing our life quality in ways we are still beginning to understand.

My journey hasn't been devoid of challenges or setbacks. I've seen how echinacea couldn't fend off every flu or how St. John's Wort wasn't a one-size-fits-all solution for mood swings. But the trials only enriched my understanding, pushing me to explore further, to fine-tune my approach, and to respect the limitations of each herb. The quest for well-being is a continual learning process, and every day brings new opportunities to grow, quite literally, in our herbal practice.

You see, personal experiences in the realm of herbal medicine are not just footnotes or anecdotal whims; they are the lifeblood of this age-old practice, a testament to its enduring relevance in modern times. As Simon Jr. Jackson, I can tell you that my relationship with herbs has grown from the roots of family tradition to blossom into a lifelong passion—a passion that transcends my own life to touch those of others, weaving a tapestry of health, comfort, and holistic wellness.

And that, dear friends, is the essence of personal experiences with herbal medicine. A voyage into the green world that isn't just about plant parts and chemical constituents but about lives touched, smiles regained, and hope continually renewed.

Continuing on, I must tell you that as time moved forward, so did my understanding of the deep interconnectedness between our health and the world of herbs. I went beyond merely treating symptoms; I started exploring herbs that could offer preventative health benefits. Take turmeric, for example. This golden root with its earthy aroma has been celebrated for its anti-inflammatory properties. When my father started experiencing the early signs of arthritis, it wasn't just pain relief we were after; we wanted to get to the root of the issue. Adding a daily regimen of turmeric tea became more than a comforting ritual; it became an act of reclaiming well-being, not just for the moment but for the years to come. Over time, he experienced a significant reduction in joint pain and improved mobility, a small victory in the broader tapestry of health.

And oh, let's talk about peppermint, shall we? A commonly underestimated herb that most of us only encounter in our toothpaste or chewing gum. My niece, Emily, had an ongoing battle with irritable bowel syndrome (IBS). Numerous visits to doctors and a cocktail of medications did offer some relief but often came with their own set of side effects. Introducing peppermint oil capsules into her diet acted like a gentle breeze clearing up a stormy sky. Emily found significant relief from abdominal pain, and the frequency of her symptoms decreased. It was an eye-opener for her and another jewel in the crown of my personal experiences with herbal medicine.

It's not just the individual herbs, but also the synergistic effects of combining different herbs that have intrigued me over the years. Consider the classic pairing of chamomile and lavender, a duo that could rival some of the greatest teams in history. While each is powerful on its own—chamomile for its soothing digestive effects and lavender for its calming influence—when combined, they offer a sort of herbal serenade that ushers you into a tranquil state of mind and body. It's like a harmonious duet sung in the language of leaves and petals.

Now, this doesn't mean my journey has been without its pitfalls. There was a time when I got overly enthusiastic about the power of garlic to improve cardiovascular health. What I didn't consider was its blood-thinning properties. A close friend who was already on anticoagulant medication decided to hop on the garlic train, and we quickly realized it wasn't the best idea. It served as a lesson about the importance of integrating herbal medicine thoughtfully, particularly if you're on specific medications or have chronic health conditions. Every herb is a tool, not a magic wand. The key is to understand when and how to use each tool properly, a lesson that comes with both study and firsthand experience.

These personal narratives are more than isolated tales of success or caution; they form the complex, richly textured fabric of a larger movement towards holistic well-being. Through my workshops and community events, I've had the privilege of witnessing many more such transformations—each unique, yet collectively building towards the same goal of empowering individuals to take control of their health naturally.

In recent years, as the conversations around mental health have rightfully gained prominence, I've been increasingly captivated by the potential of herbs like St. John's Wort and ashwagandha. These aren't just plants; they're silent warriors, standing tall and rooted in their healing capabilities. They don't promise an overnight cure, but they do offer something perhaps even more valuable—a partnership, a commitment to walk alongside you as you navigate the peaks and valleys of your emotional landscape.

To sum up, my name is Simon Jr. Jackson, and my lifelong exploration of herbal medicine has been more than a scholarly pursuit. It's been a journey marked by discovery, bonding, challenges, and above all, an enduring respect for the wisdom encapsulated in each leaf, root, and petal. From the innocent days of sage tea for sore throats to the mature understanding of herbal combinations and their nuanced effects, each chapter has enriched my life and those of the people around me. It's a journey I'm grateful for, and one that continues to unfold in exciting, enlightening ways. Because, in the grand scheme of things, aren't we all just students sitting in the verdant classroom of Mother Nature, eager to learn the ancient yet ever-new lessons she has to teach us?

Clinical Insights: What the Research Says

As Simon Jr. Jackson, my story so far has been a blend of anecdotal experiences and personal relationships with the herbs I've come to deeply respect. However, I'm keenly aware that personal narratives, while compelling, are just one facet of the complex gemstone that is herbal medicine. To fully appreciate its dimensions, we need to turn our attention to what might be considered the 'science' behind the 'magic'—the realm of clinical insights and research.

Now, it's no secret that herbal medicine, despite its ancient lineage, has often been regarded with skepticism by the mainstream medical community. However, the tides have been turning, and scientific validation is lending credibility to what many traditional cultures have known for millennia. Over the past few decades, rigorous research has begun to unearth the pharmacological bases for the effectiveness of numerous herbs, thereby bridging the gap between folklore and evidence-based medicine.

Take, for instance, the herb turmeric that I mentioned earlier, which my father uses for his arthritis. Curcumin, the active compound in turmeric, has undergone extensive research, not just for its anti-inflammatory effects but also for its potential role in cancer prevention, wound healing, and even as a neuroprotective agent. Studies using controlled groups and scientific methods have confirmed the beneficial effects of curcumin, which has propelled turmeric from the spice shelf to the supplement aisle in health food stores. It's as if turmeric, an age-old remedy, has gotten a new badge of honor, stamped by modern science.

Similarly, the peppermint oil capsules that have been such a blessing for Emily, my niece, weren't just a random choice. Research has indicated that the menthol in peppermint oil can effectively relax the muscles of the gastrointestinal tract, making it a viable treatment for IBS symptoms. Clinical trials have provided quantifiable data, paving the way for peppermint oil's acceptance into more traditional treatment plans.

And let's not forget the venerable St. John's Wort, which has become something of a poster child for herbal antidepressants. While the herb has been on the periphery for a long time, it has received its fair share of scientific scrutiny. Meta-analyses comparing the efficacy of St. John's Wort with standard antidepressants suggest that the herb can be as effective for mild to moderate depression, with fewer side effects. However, it's important to note that these studies also indicate that St. John's Wort can interact with various medications, underscoring the necessity for professional medical guidance.

This emerging body of research not only supports the validity of herbal treatments but also helps standardize dosages, identifies contraindications, and even inspires new lines of pharmacological inquiry. It's like a symphony where ancient wisdom and modern science are different sections of the orchestra, each contributing its unique sound to a harmonious composition. Sure, there are still some dissonant notes and gaps in our understanding, but as each study builds on its predecessors, a clearer, more nuanced picture begins to emerge.

Moreover, research also brings a degree of caution and balance to the enthusiasm surrounding herbal medicine. For every study that finds positive results, there may be another that reveals limitations or potential risks, reminding us that herbal medicine isn't a panacea but a continually evolving field that requires both respect and scrutiny.

It's a thrilling time to be involved in this space. As someone who's had a lifelong relationship with herbs, witnessing this scientific validation feels like watching a close friend receive a well-deserved award. It enriches not just my personal practice but also contributes to a broader, more holistic understanding of health. It serves as both a vindication of past wisdom and a roadmap for future discoveries.

In essence, my experiences and observations, when viewed through the lens of scientific research, take on a new dimension, one that is both gratifying and humbling. They remind me that while the path of herbal medicine may be strewn with leaves, roots, and petals, it also intersects with the highways of modern science. And as someone deeply invested in both, I can't help but feel excited about what lies at that intersection, for it's there that we truly find the promise of a more integrated, more compassionate, and more holistic approach to well-being.

Appendix A: Glossary of Herbal Terms

Let's switch gears a bit and delve into a glossary that serves as your herbal roadmap. A handy reference, if you will, for all those botanical names, tricky terminologies, and herbal jargon that can make your eyes glaze over. But don't worry, I'm not about to drop a Latin textbook on you. Think of this more like your pocket guide, a trusted companion for your herbal journey.

Adaptogen: Let's start with a term that's been creating some buzz lately. Adaptogens are herbs that help your body adapt to stress. Think of them as your body's personal cheerleading squad, encouraging you to handle life's curveballs with grace. Examples include ashwagandha, holy basil, and ginseng.

Antibacterial: These herbs help fight off bacterial infections. Garlic is a potent antibacterial you probably have in your kitchen right now.

Antispasmodic: Suffering from muscle cramps or spasms? Antispasmodic herbs help alleviate those symptoms. Cramp bark is your straightforward, no-nonsense friend here.

Anthraquinones: These are naturally occurring compounds found in certain herbs that often have laxative effects. Aloe vera is a well-known example.

Astringent: Nope, it's not just for skin toners. An astringent herb has the quality of tightening tissues. Imagine drawing the curtains closed on a sunny day; that's what these herbs do, often minimizing discharges like diarrhea or bleeding. Witch hazel is a popular astringent.

Alterative: These herbs are like the housecleaners of your bloodstream. They help improve nutrient absorption and waste elimination. Burdock is a classic example.

Antipyretic: Herbs that help reduce fever. Elderflower and yarrow might be in your anti-fever toolkit.

Antiviral: Herbs that help fight viral infections, such as echinacea and elderberry.

Astringent: These herbs tighten tissues and can help manage issues like diarrhea or skin conditions. Witch hazel is a popular one.

Anti-emetic: Feeling queasy? Anti-emetics like ginger can help prevent or relieve nausea and vomiting.

Bitter: These herbs have a bitter flavor and are often used to stimulate digestion. Gentian is one you might hear about often in this category.

Carminative: Sounds like a type of gemstone, doesn't it? But carminative herbs are those that help with digestion and relieve gas. Imagine them as your post-Thanksgiving dinner saviors. Think peppermint and ginger.

Cholagogue: Aiding the gallbladder in bile secretion, herbs like milk thistle can be helpful.

Choleretic: Similar to cholagogues, these herbs stimulate the liver to produce more bile, but they don't necessarily aid in its secretion. Turmeric is one example.

Decoction: Not to be confused with its cousin infusion, a decoction is made by boiling the tougher parts of the herb like roots and barks. It's like slow-cooking a hearty stew, extracting as much goodness as possible.

Diuretic: These are the herbs that help your body shed excess water by increasing urine production. Dandelion and parsley are your go-to natural diuretics.

Demulcent: Think of these herbs as the internal moisturizers. They soothe and protect inflamed or irritated tissue. Slippery elm is your go-to.

Expectorant: These herbs help clear mucus from the respiratory system. Mullein is a star player here.

Emollient: Topical herbs that soften and soothe the skin, like calendula

Emmenagogue: No, it's not a mystical incantation, though it might seem like one. Emmenagogues are herbs that stimulate menstrual flow, serving as herbal allies for women. Examples include parsley and yarrow.

Expectorant: These are the herbs you want on your team during a nasty cough. They help clear mucus from the respiratory system. If they were a gadget, they'd be your vacuum cleaner for the lungs. Herbs like mullein and elecampane serve this role.

Febrifuge: Herbs that reduce fever but are not necessarily antipyretic; they work by promoting sweating. Boneset is one such herb.

Galactagogue: For nursing mothers, these herbs like fenugreek can help increase milk supply.

Hepatic: These herbs support liver health, like milk thistle and dandelion root.

Mucilage: Sounds like something from a sci-fi movie, but it's less scary than it sounds. Mucilaginous herbs like marshmallow root form a gooey substance when mixed with water, soothing irritated tissues. Imagine them as your body's internal band-aid.

Nervine: These are herbs specifically geared toward supporting the nervous system. If your nerves are frazzled, nervines like lemon balm and valerian are there to sing them a calming lullaby.

Nootropic: Cognitive enhancers like ginkgo biloba fall under this category.

Parturient: Herbs that assist in childbirth by strengthening and toning the uterine muscles. Raspberry leaf is commonly used.

Pectoral: Herbs beneficial for chest and respiratory issues, like mullein.

Rubefacient: Topical herbs that increase blood flow and can warm the skin, like cayenne pepper.

Saponins: These are phytochemicals found in many plants that produce a soap-like foam when shaken in water. They have various health benefits and can be found in herbs like ginseng.

Tonic: These herbs promote overall well-being and health, such as nettle and ginseng.

Vasoconstrictor: These herbs like yarrow can constrict blood vessels and may be useful for conditions like varicose veins.

Vasodilator: The opposite of vasoconstrictors, these herbs expand blood vessels. Garlic is a prime example.

Vermifuge: These herbs help expel intestinal parasites. Wormwood is a classic choice.

Vulnerary: These are the medics of the herbal world, aiding in the healing of wounds. Comfrey and calendula, step right up!

Volatile oils: Also known as essential oils, these are the aromatic compounds found in plants. They're like the plant's perfume, only more therapeutic. Lavender and eucalyptus oils are popular examples.

Appendix B: Herb Profiles

Here we are, the final stretch of our herbal journey, landing at the doorway of Appendix B: Herb Profiles. Now, this isn't just a catalog or a mere list, no sir! This is more like your herbal rolodex, your go-to directory, and the resource you'll find yourself flipping back to time and time again, whether you're a novice herbalist or someone who's been steeped—pun intended—in the world of herbs for years.

Aloe Vera
Identification: Aloe Vera plants have thick, fleshy, spiky leaves that contain a clear gel.
Growing Conditions: Thrives in well-drained soil and bright, indirect sunlight. Sensitive to frost.
Harvesting Time: Best to harvest the outer leaves as the plant matures, generally after 8-12 months.
Medicinal Uses: Used topically for skin conditions like burns and cuts, and orally for digestive issues.
Active Components: Contains aloin, barbaloin, and aloe-emodin among others.
Dosage and Preparation: Aloe gel can be applied directly to the skin. Oral doses vary but should be taken under the guidance of a healthcare provider.
Safety Protocols and Storage: Not recommended for pregnant women or those with kidney issues when taken orally. Store gel in a cool, dark place.

Ashwagandha
Identification: Small shrub with yellow flowers and red fruit. The roots are the primary medicinal part.
Growing Conditions: Prefers dry regions and can tolerate poor soil quality.
Harvesting Time: Roots are harvested in late autumn or early winter.
Medicinal Uses: Known for reducing stress and boosting the immune system.
Active Components: Contains withanolides, alkaloids, and choline.
Dosage and Preparation: Commonly taken as a powder, tincture, or capsule. Typical dose ranges from 300mg to 500mg.
Safety Protocols and Storage: Generally safe but should be avoided during pregnancy. Store in a dry place.

Astragalus Root
Identification: A perennial plant in the legume family. The roots are harvested for medicinal use.
Growing Conditions: Prefers sandy, well-drained soil and full sun.
Harvesting Time: Roots are harvested from 4-year-old plants in spring or fall.
Medicinal Uses: Often used to boost the immune system and improve cardiovascular health.
Active Components: Contains flavonoids, saponins, and polysaccharides.

Dosage and Preparation: Typically taken as a capsule, tincture, or tea.

Safety Protocols and Storage: Generally safe but should be avoided if you have certain immune disorders. Store in a dry place.

Basil

Identification: Green, leafy plant with a strong, sweet aroma. Purple or white flowers depending on the variety.

Growing Conditions: Prefers well-drained soil and lots of sunlight.

Harvesting Time: Early morning is the best time, usually just before flowering for highest oil content.

Medicinal Uses: Used for anxiety, stress, and anti-inflammatory purposes.

Active Components: Contains essential oils like eugenol, flavonoids, and antioxidants.

Dosage and Preparation: Can be used fresh, as an essential oil, or dried.

Safety Protocols and Storage: Generally safe in food amounts. Store in a cool, dark place.

Black Cohosh

Identification: Tall perennial plant with a large, branched rootstock. It has white flowers.

Growing Conditions: Prefers woodland conditions with well-drained soil.

Harvesting Time: Roots are harvested in the fall after the plant has finished flowering.

Medicinal Uses: Mainly used for menstrual and menopausal symptoms.

Active Components: Contains triterpenoid saponins, particularly actein and cimicifugoside.

Dosage and Preparation: Often taken as a tablet, capsule, or tincture. Follow healthcare provider's recommendations.

Safety Protocols and Storage: Not recommended for pregnant or lactating women. Store in a cool, dry place.

Burdock Root

Identification: A biennial plant with large, heart-shaped leaves and purple or pink flowers. The long taproot is used medicinally.

Growing Conditions: Grows best in well-drained, deep soils and requires moderate sunlight.

Harvesting Time: Best harvested in the fall of the first year or spring of the second year.

Medicinal Uses: Known for its blood-purifying qualities and is often used for skin conditions like acne.

Active Components: Rich in polyphenols and fiber.

Dosage and Preparation: Usually consumed as a tea, tincture, or capsules.

Safety Protocols and Storage: Generally considered safe, but pregnant and nursing women should avoid. Store in a dry, cool place.

Calendula (Marigold)

Identification: These plants have bright orange or yellow flowers. It's the petals that are used for medicinal purposes.

Growing Conditions: Loves well-drained soil and full to partial sun.

Harvesting Time: Harvest flowers as they open during the growing season.

Medicinal Uses: Widely used for skin conditions, to promote wound healing, and as an anti-inflammatory.

Active Components: Contains flavonoids and carotenoids.

Dosage and Preparation: Often used as an oil or tea. It can also be made into creams or salves.

Safety Protocols and Storage: Generally considered safe but avoid during pregnancy. Store the petals away from light to preserve color and potency.

Cayenne Pepper
Identification: This is a type of chili pepper, used commonly in powder form.
Growing Conditions: Prefers warm, well-drained soil and plenty of sunlight.
Harvesting Time: Best when pods are mature and have turned bright red.
Medicinal Uses: Known for boosting metabolism and reducing pain.
Active Components: Contains capsaicin, which is the component responsible for its heat.
Dosage and Preparation: Can be used as a spice, in capsule form, or as a cream for topical application.
Safety Protocols and Storage: Use with caution if you have gastrointestinal issues. Store in a cool, dark place.

Chamomile
Identification: Chamomile has daisy-like flowers with a sweet, apple-like scent.
Growing Conditions: Prefers open, sandy soil in sun or partial shade.
Harvesting Time: The flowers are harvested when fully open, generally in late summer.
Medicinal Uses: Widely used to treat insomnia, gastrointestinal issues, and skin conditions.
Active Components: Contains flavonoids, particularly apigenin.
Dosage and Preparation: Commonly consumed as tea but also available in capsules and tinctures.
Safety Protocols and Storage: Generally safe but can cause allergic reactions in some people. Store in a cool, dry place.

Chickweed
Identification: This is a low-growing plant with small white flowers.
Growing Conditions: Grows in a variety of conditions but prefers moist soils.
Harvesting Time: Best harvested in the spring when the plants are vibrant but before flowering.
Medicinal Uses: Used for skin conditions and as a mild diuretic.
Active Components: Rich in flavonoids and saponins.
Dosage and Preparation: Can be eaten fresh in salads, or used as a tea or salve.
Safety Protocols and Storage: Generally considered safe but consume in moderate amounts. Store in a cool, dry place.

Cilantro
Identification: This popular culinary herb has flat, feathery leaves and produces tiny white flowers.
Growing Conditions: Enjoys well-drained soil and moderate sunlight. Be careful; it bolts easily, meaning it'll go to seed rather quickly.
Harvesting Time: Best harvested just before it flowers, usually late spring or early summer.
Medicinal Uses: Known for its detoxifying properties and is also used to combat bad breath.
Active Components: Contains phytonutrients, flavonoids, and phenolic compounds.
Dosage and Preparation: Typically consumed fresh in culinary dishes but also available in tincture and supplement forms.
Safety Protocols and Storage: Generally safe for most people. Store fresh leaves in the refrigerator and dried forms in a cool, dry place.

Cinnamon
Identification: Cinnamon is the bark of trees in the Cinnamomum family.
Growing Conditions: Prefers a tropical climate and well-drained soil.
Harvesting Time: The bark is harvested during the rainy season when more pliable.
Medicinal Uses: Commonly used for gastrointestinal issues and has been studied for its potential in lowering blood sugar.
Active Components: Contains cinnamaldehyde, which gives it its flavor and aroma.
Dosage and Preparation: Used as a spice in cooking or as a supplement.
Safety Protocols and Storage: Excessive amounts may be toxic, especially for those with liver issues. Store in a cool, dry place.

Comfrey
Identification: Has broad leaves and bell-shaped purple, cream, or pink flowers.
Growing Conditions: Thrives in damp, grassy locations.
Harvesting Time: Leaves are harvested before flowering, usually in late spring.
Medicinal Uses: Traditionally used for wound healing and bone fractures.
Active Components: Contains allantoin and rosmarinic acid.
Dosage and Preparation: Commonly used in topical preparations like creams and ointments.
Safety Protocols and Storage: Not recommended for internal use due to toxicity concerns. Store in a cool, dry place.

Dandelion
Identification: A common weed with bright yellow flowers and a rosette of leaves at the base.
Growing Conditions: Extremely hardy and can grow in a variety of conditions.
Harvesting Time: Leaves are best harvested in the spring, roots in the fall.
Medicinal Uses: Used for liver detoxification and as a diuretic.
Active Components: Rich in vitamins and minerals, including vitamin A, K, and iron.
Dosage and Preparation: Can be consumed as a tea, tincture, or even fresh in salads.
Safety Protocols and Storage: Generally considered safe but may interact with certain medications. Store in a cool, dry place.

Echinacea
Identification: Known for its beautiful, purple coneflowers.
Growing Conditions: Prefers well-drained soil and full to partial sunlight.
Harvesting Time: The roots are harvested in the fall of the plant's third or fourth year.
Medicinal Uses: Most commonly used to boost the immune system.
Active Components: Contains phenols, alkamides, and flavonoids.
Dosage and Preparation: Commonly consumed as a tea or tincture but also available in capsule form.
Safety Protocols and Storage: Generally safe but can cause allergic reactions in some people. Store in a cool, dry place.

Elderberry
Identification: This shrub produces dark purple-black berries and has clusters of small white flowers.
Growing Conditions: Prefers well-drained, loamy soil and full to partial sun.
Harvesting Time: Berries are ready for harvest late summer to early fall.
Medicinal Uses: Highly esteemed for its antiviral properties, particularly against the common cold and flu.
Active Components: Rich in flavonoids and antioxidants.
Dosage and Preparation: Commonly used in syrups, teas, and lozenges.
Safety Protocols and Storage: Raw berries are toxic and must be cooked. Store in a cool, dark place.

Fennel
Identification: Feathery leaves and produces yellow flowers. Seeds, leaves, and roots are all used.
Growing Conditions: Grows best in dry soils near the coast or on riverbanks.
Harvesting Time: Late summer when the seeds have matured.
Medicinal Uses: Known for its digestive benefits and also acts as a mild diuretic.
Active Components: Contains flavonoids, essential oils, and coumarins.
Dosage and Preparation: Used in cooking, teas, and tinctures.
Safety Protocols and Storage: Generally considered safe but may interact with certain medications. Store in a cool, dry place.

Fenugreek
Identification: Features light green leaves and produces slender, long pods containing seeds.
Growing Conditions: Thrives in full sun and well-drained soil.
Harvesting Time: Ready to harvest 4-8 months after planting.
Medicinal Uses: Often used for digestive issues and to boost milk production in breastfeeding mothers.
Active Components: Rich in proteins, fibers, and other phytonutrients.
Dosage and Preparation: Used as seeds, powder, or in capsule form.
Safety Protocols and Storage: Can lower blood sugar; those on diabetes medication should consult a healthcare provider. Store in a cool, dry place.

Garlic
Identification: Well-known for its bulb that's divided into cloves.
Growing Conditions: Prefers full sun and well-drained soil.
Harvesting Time: Late spring or early summer when the leaves begin to yellow.
Medicinal Uses: Widely known for its antimicrobial properties and its benefits for cardiovascular health.
Active Components: Contains allicin, which has potent medicinal properties.
Dosage and Preparation: Consumed in raw or cooked form, and available as a supplement.
Safety Protocols and Storage: Generally safe but consult your healthcare provider if you're taking blood thinners. Store in a cool, dry place.

Ginkgo Biloba
Identification: Recognizable for its fan-shaped leaves.
Growing Conditions: Very hardy and can withstand various soil types and environmental conditions.
Harvesting Time: Late summer or early fall for leaves, and fall for seeds.
Medicinal Uses: Mainly used for cognitive function and circulatory issues.
Active Components: Contains flavonoids and terpenoids, which are antioxidants.
Dosage and Preparation: Usually consumed as a supplement or extract.
Safety Protocols and Storage: Consult a healthcare provider if you're on medications like anticoagulants. Store in a cool, dry place.

Ginseng
Identification: Ginseng is identified by its fleshy roots, which sometimes look a bit like a human figure.
Growing Conditions: Prefers well-drained, humus-rich soils in the shade.
Harvesting Time: Typically, the older the root, the more potent its medicinal qualities. Most are harvested after 4-6 years.
Medicinal Uses: Known for its adaptogenic properties, it helps with stress, enhances physical performance, and can aid in improving cognitive function.
Active Components: Contains ginsenosides, which are thought to be the active compounds.
Dosage and Preparation: Available in various forms, including as a tea, tincture, or capsule.
Safety Protocols and Storage: Generally considered safe but consult your healthcare provider if you're pregnant or on medications like blood thinners. Store in a cool, dry place.

Goldenseal
Identification: Recognizable by its thick, yellow root and purplish stem.
Growing Conditions: Prefers shady, moist, and wooded areas.
Harvesting Time: Late summer to early fall.
Medicinal Uses: Commonly used for digestive issues and skin disorders.
Active Components: Contains berberine, a powerful antimicrobial compound.
Dosage and Preparation: Often used as a tincture, tea, or in capsule form.
Safety Protocols and Storage: Not recommended for pregnant or breastfeeding women. Store in a cool, dry place.

Hawthorn
Identification: A tree that produces red berries and has thorny branches.
Growing Conditions: Adaptable to many soil types but prefers full sun.
Harvesting Time: Late spring for flowers and late summer for berries.
Medicinal Uses: Primarily known for its cardiovascular benefits, such as lowering blood pressure and cholesterol levels.
Active Components: Rich in antioxidants like flavonoids.
Dosage and Preparation: Consumed as a tea, tincture, or in capsule form.
Safety Protocols and Storage: Consult a healthcare provider if you're on heart medications. Store in a cool, dry place.

Holy Basil (Tulsi)
Identification: Similar in appearance to regular basil but with a more purple stem.
Growing Conditions: Thrives in full sun and well-drained soil.
Harvesting Time: Early morning or late afternoon for maximum essential oil content.
Medicinal Uses: Known for its adaptogenic, antibacterial, and anti-inflammatory properties.
Active Components: Contains eugenol, a potent essential oil.
Dosage and Preparation: Used in teas, tinctures, and also as a culinary herb.
Safety Protocols and Storage: Generally considered safe but consult a healthcare provider if pregnant. Store in a cool, dry place.

Horehound
Identification: Features crinkly leaves that resemble mint and produces small white flowers.
Growing Conditions: Prefers dry, sandy soil and full sun to partial shade.
Harvesting Time: Late spring to early summer.
Medicinal Uses: Most commonly used for respiratory issues, like coughs and asthma.
Active Components: Contains marrubiin, which is thought to be responsible for its medicinal properties.
Dosage and Preparation: Used in cough syrups, teas, and lozenges.
Safety Protocols and Storage: Generally safe but high doses can cause stomach upset. Store in a cool, dry place.

Juniper
Identification: Juniper is a small shrub or tree with needle-like leaves and blueish berries.
Growing Conditions: Prefers well-drained soils and can handle dry and rocky conditions. Loves full sun.
Harvesting Time: Berries can be picked from late summer through fall.
Medicinal Uses: Used primarily for digestive issues and urinary tract infections.
Active Components: Contains a variety of essential oils and flavonoids.
Dosage and Preparation: Used in teas, tinctures, and essential oils.
Safety Protocols and Storage: Not recommended for those who are pregnant, nursing, or have kidney issues. Store berries and oil in a cool, dark place.

Lavender
Identification: Known for its beautiful purple flowers and iconic scent.
Growing Conditions: Loves well-drained soil and lots of sunshine.
Harvesting Time: Mid to late summer when flowers are in full bloom.
Medicinal Uses: Lavender is famous for its calming effects, and it's also an antiseptic.
Active Components: Rich in essential oils like linalool.
Dosage and Preparation: Can be used in teas, oils, and even culinary dishes.
Safety Protocols and Storage: Generally considered safe but can be potent, so use in moderation. Store in a cool, dark place.

Lemon Balm
Identification: A mint family member, this herb has light green leaves with a lemony scent.
Growing Conditions: Enjoys well-drained soil and partial shade.
Harvesting Time: Late spring to early fall.
Medicinal Uses: Known for its calming effects and is good for indigestion.

Active Components: Contains terpenes which are responsible for its calming effects.
Dosage and Preparation: Popular as a tea or tincture.
Safety Protocols and Storage: Generally safe but check with healthcare provider if you're pregnant or nursing. Store dried leaves in an airtight container.

Licorice Root

Identification: Licorice is a woody plant with light, feathery leaves.
Growing Conditions: Prefers well-drained soils and full sun.
Harvesting Time: Roots are usually harvested in the fall.
Medicinal Uses: Often used for digestive issues and respiratory problems.
Active Components: Contains glycyrrhizin, which is many times sweeter than sugar.
Dosage and Preparation: Available in teas, tinctures, and capsules.
Safety Protocols and Storage: Not recommended for those with hypertension or pregnant women. Store in a cool, dark place.

Marshmallow Root

Identification: Has pale pink flowers and large, soft leaves.
Growing Conditions: Enjoys moist, well-drained soil and partial sun.
Harvesting Time: Roots are harvested in late fall.
Medicinal Uses: Used for soothing mucous membranes, such as those in the throat and stomach.
Active Components: Rich in mucilage, which gives it its soothing properties.
Dosage and Preparation: Commonly used in teas and tinctures.
Safety Protocols and Storage: Generally considered safe but consult your healthcare provider if you're pregnant or nursing. Store in a cool, dark place.

Milk Thistle

Identification: Recognizable by its spiky, purple flowers and marbled leaves.
Growing Conditions: Enjoys full sun and well-drained soil but is pretty resilient and can tolerate drought.
Harvesting Time: Late spring to early summer for the leaves and late summer for the seeds.
Medicinal Uses: Famed for its liver-protective qualities.
Active Components: Contains a compound called silymarin.
Dosage and Preparation: Often taken as a supplement, tincture, or even in tea form.
Safety Protocols and Storage: Generally well-tolerated but consult a healthcare provider if you're pregnant, nursing, or on other medications. Store in a cool, dark place.

Motherwort

Identification: This plant has a tall stem covered in downy hairs, and small, pink to lavender flowers.
Growing Conditions: Flexible, growing well in both sun and shade and a variety of soil types.
Harvesting Time: Mid to late summer.
Medicinal Uses: Often used for anxiety, and some people find it useful for heart issues like palpitations.
Active Components: Rich in alkaloids and tannins.
Dosage and Preparation: Commonly used in tinctures and teas.
Safety Protocols and Storage: Not for pregnant or nursing women. Store in a cool, dark place.

Mullein

Identification: Tall, with a rosette of woolly leaves at the base and a single stem ending in a spike of yellow flowers.

Growing Conditions: Prefers well-drained soil and full sun but is highly adaptable.

Harvesting Time: Late summer.

Medicinal Uses: Often used for respiratory issues, including bronchitis and asthma.

Active Components: Contains a variety of flavonoids and other compounds.

Dosage and Preparation: Generally used as a tea or tincture.

Safety Protocols and Storage: Generally considered safe. Store in an airtight container in a cool, dark place.

Nettle

Identification: Also known as stinging nettle, it has small, almost heart-shaped leaves and can indeed sting if touched!

Growing Conditions: Thrives in rich soil and partial shade.

Harvesting Time: Early to mid-spring for the leaves, later for the seeds.

Medicinal Uses: Known for anti-inflammatory properties and often used for arthritis and allergies.

Active Components: Rich in a variety of nutrients, including vitamins and minerals.

Dosage and Preparation: Available in tea form, as a supplement, or even as an ingredient in food.

Safety Protocols and Storage: Wear gloves when harvesting! Store dried leaves in an airtight container in a cool, dark place.

Oregano

Identification: Small, spade-shaped, green leaves on a woody stem, sometimes with tiny purple flowers.

Growing Conditions: Loves well-drained soil and full sun.

Harvesting Time: Late spring through early fall.

Medicinal Uses: Not just for pizza! Known for its antimicrobial properties.

Active Components: Contains compounds like carvacrol and thymol.

Dosage and Preparation: Used as an essential oil, tincture, or even just added to food.

Safety Protocols and Storage: Generally safe, but the oil can be potent, so dilution is advised. Store in a cool, dark place.

Passionflower

Identification: Known for its intricate, purple flowers that almost resemble little clock faces.

Growing Conditions: Prefers full sun to partial shade and well-drained soil.

Harvesting Time: Late summer to early fall for the flowers, while leaves can be harvested throughout the growing season.

Medicinal Uses: Often used as a natural sedative or to treat anxiety.

Active Components: Contains flavonoids that are thought to induce relaxation.

Dosage and Preparation: Generally consumed as a tea or tincture.

Safety Protocols and Storage: Be cautious if you're on other sedatives or are pregnant. Store dried herbs in a cool, dark place.

Peppermint

Identification: Easily identifiable by its square stem and its dark green, serrated leaves.
Growing Conditions: Thrives in moist, shaded places but can also grow in full sun.
Harvesting Time: Late spring to early autumn.
Medicinal Uses: A go-to for digestive issues and headaches.
Active Components: The star here is menthol.
Dosage and Preparation: Commonly enjoyed as a tea, essential oil, or tincture.
Safety Protocols and Storage: Fairly safe but can interfere with certain medications. Store in a cool, dark place.

Plantain Leaf

Identification: Has broad, oval leaves and may display small, inconspicuous flowers.
Growing Conditions: Remarkably adaptable, thriving in both poor, dry soils and richer, moist soils.
Harvesting Time: Spring and summer are optimal.
Medicinal Uses: Effective for skin conditions, minor wounds, and insect bites.
Active Components: Rich in tannins and mucilage.
Dosage and Preparation: Often applied as a poultice or taken as a tea or tincture.
Safety Protocols and Storage: Generally safe. Store dried leaves in an airtight container in a cool, dark place.

Red Clover

Identification: Known for its pinkish-purple flowers and trifoliate leaves.
Growing Conditions: Prefers loamy soil and full sun to partial shade.
Harvesting Time: Late spring to early summer.
Medicinal Uses: Often used to treat skin conditions and for its phytoestrogen content.
Active Components: Contains isoflavones.
Dosage and Preparation: Generally consumed as a tea or tincture.
Safety Protocols and Storage: Avoid if you're pregnant or have hormone-sensitive conditions. Store dried flowers in a cool, dark place.

Rosemary

Identification: It's a woody shrub with needle-like leaves and blue flowers.
Growing Conditions: Loves the sun and prefers well-drained soil.
Harvesting Time: Spring and summer for the fresh leaves.
Medicinal Uses: Besides flavoring your focaccia, it's known for enhancing memory and circulation.
Active Components: Contains compounds like rosmarinic acid and various antioxidants.
Dosage and Preparation: Used as an essential oil, tincture, or simply as a culinary herb.
Safety Protocols and Storage: Generally safe, but high doses can lead to complications. Store in a cool, dark place.

Sage

Identification: Think silvery green leaves and purple, blue, or even white flowers.
Growing Conditions: Enjoys full sun and well-drained soil.
Harvesting Time: Late spring through summer is ideal.
Medicinal Uses: Great for sore throats, digestive issues, and even improving memory.
Active Components: Contains flavonoids, phenolic acids, and more.

Dosage and Preparation: Commonly consumed as a tea or as an essential oil.

Safety Protocols and Storage: Generally safe but should be avoided in large doses or by pregnant women. Store in a cool, dark place.

Skullcap
Identification: Small, tube-like blue flowers and heart-shaped leaves.
Growing Conditions: Prefers partial shade and moist, well-drained soil.
Harvesting Time: Late spring to early autumn.
Medicinal Uses: Known for its calming effects and often used for anxiety and insomnia.
Active Components: Contains flavonoids and essential oils.
Dosage and Preparation: Generally taken as a tea or tincture.
Safety Protocols and Storage: Be cautious if you're already on sedatives. Store dried herbs in a cool, dark place.

Slippery Elm
Identification: The inner bark is the useful part, which is kind of reddish-brown.
Growing Conditions: Prefers slightly acidic to neutral soils and partial to full sun.
Harvesting Time: Late autumn to early winter for the inner bark.
Medicinal Uses: Excellent for sore throats, coughs, and digestive issues.
Active Components: Mucilage is the star player here.
Dosage and Preparation: Used in teas, lozenges, and capsules.
Safety Protocols and Storage: Generally safe but consult healthcare providers if you're pregnant. Store in a cool, dry place.

St. John's Wort
Identification: Yellow flowers and opposite leaves that have tiny translucent dots.
Growing Conditions: Loves full sun and sandy soil.
Harvesting Time: Mid to late summer.
Medicinal Uses: Primarily known for treating depression and mood swings.
Active Components: Hypericin is the main component.
Dosage and Preparation: Consumed as a tea, capsule, or tincture.
Safety Protocols and Storage: Can interfere with a lot of medications. Store in a cool, dark place.

Thyme
Identification: Tiny lilac or pink flowers and small, fragrant, greenish-gray leaves.
Growing Conditions: Full sun and well-drained soil.
Harvesting Time: Late spring through summer.
Medicinal Uses: Great for respiratory issues, coughs, and bronchitis.
Active Components: Thymol is the main one.
Dosage and Preparation: Commonly used as a tea, tincture, or even in a bath.
Safety Protocols and Storage: Generally safe but large doses can cause digestive issues. Store in a cool, dark place.

Turmeric
Identification: Vibrant orange-yellow root, often ground into a powder.
Growing Conditions: Loves warm, humid climates and well-drained soil.

Harvesting Time: About 8 to 10 months after planting when the leaves and stem start to brown and dry.
Medicinal Uses: Anti-inflammatory, great for joint pain, and can even brighten your mood.
Active Components: Curcumin is the superstar here.
Dosage and Preparation: Often used in teas, capsules, or even as a spice in food.
Safety Protocols and Storage: Generally safe, but high doses can cause stomach upset. Store in a cool, dark place.

Valerian
Identification: Think tall, upright stems with umbrella-like heads and sweetly scented pink or white flowers.
Growing Conditions: Enjoys well-drained soil and prefers full sun to partial shade.
Harvesting Time: Late summer to early autumn for the roots.
Medicinal Uses: Fantastic for sleep disorders and dealing with stress.
Active Components: Contains valerenic acid, among others.
Dosage and Preparation: Used in teas, tinctures, or capsules.
Safety Protocols and Storage: Generally safe, but consult your doctor if you're on medication. Store roots in a cool, dry place.

White Willow Bark
Identification: Bark is grey-brown and cracked, leaves are long and thin.
Growing Conditions: Likes moist and loamy soil and full sun to partial shade.
Harvesting Time: Early spring for the bark.
Medicinal Uses: Pain relief, especially for headaches and lower back pain.
Active Components: The key is salicin, which your body turns into salicylic acid.
Dosage and Preparation: Usually consumed as a tincture or tea.
Safety Protocols and Storage: Use cautiously if you're allergic to aspirin. Store bark in a cool, dark place.

Yarrow
Identification: White or light-colored flower clusters on top of long, thin stalks.
Growing Conditions: Very adaptable but prefers well-drained soil and full sun.
Harvesting Time: Late spring through early autumn.
Medicinal Uses: Good for wounds, infections, and even for digestive issues.
Active Components: Contains flavonoids, tannins, and volatile oils.
Dosage and Preparation: Used fresh, dried, or as a tincture or tea.
Safety Protocols and Storage: Generally safe but should be avoided by pregnant women. Store in a cool, dark place.

Conclusion

In our journey through "The Lost Herbal Medicine Bible," we've delved deep into the annals of time, rediscovering the profound knowledge our ancestors held about the natural world. From the soil beneath our feet to the very essence of our souls, the power of plants and herbs to heal, nourish, and rejuvenate has been a testament to the intricate connections we share with Mother Earth.

The art of crafting essential oils, tinctures, infusions, and even antibiotics from these natural sources is not just a mere skill—it's a legacy, a bridge that connects us to a time when humanity lived in harmony with nature. In an age of synthetic drugs and fast-paced lifestyles, this book serves as a reminder that sometimes, the best remedies are those crafted with our own hands, guided by the wisdom of generations past.

Moreover, as we've learned, herbal medicine is not just about physical healing. It's about a holistic approach to health, one that encompasses the mind, body, and spirit. When we take a tincture or inhale the aroma of an essential oil, we're not just treating a symptom; we're inviting balance, harmony, and vitality into our lives.

In conclusion, "The Lost Herbal Medicine Bible" is more than just a guide. It's a call to action—a plea to reconnect with the natural world, to respect the ancient wisdom of herbal remedies, and to take charge of our own well-being. As we close this chapter, let's carry forward the lessons learned, cherishing the age-old practices, and ensuring that the legacy of herbal medicine thrives for generations to come.

May the earth's bounty continue to nurture your body and soul, guiding you towards a life of health, balance, and profound connection.

Bonus

Dear reader,

Thank you for embarking on this enlightening journey through "The Lost Herbal Medicine Bible." While the written word provides a wealth of knowledge, sometimes, seeing is believing. If you wish to delve deeper and witness firsthand the art and science of herbal preparations, we have a special treat for you!

Simply scan the QR code below with your smartphone or tablet. This will lead you to a series of comprehensive video tutorials, where experts demonstrate the nuances of crafting essential oils, tinctures, infusions, and more. From the selection of the right herbs to the intricacies of the extraction process, these videos are designed to enhance your understanding and skills in the realm of herbal medicine.

@YOURHEALINGHERBS

We hope these tutorials serve as a valuable companion to the knowledge you've gained from this book. Here's to a hands-on, immersive experience in the world of herbs!

Warmly, Simon.

Made in United States
Troutdale, OR
08/02/2024

21716762R00064